W9-AOU-589

THE Men'sHealth Diet

THE 6-WEEK PLAN TO FLATTEN YOUR STOMACH & FUEL YOUR MUSCLES

STEPHEN PERRINE

With ADAM BORNSTEIN, HEATHER HURLOCK,
and the EDITORS of *Men's Health*

RODALE

Rodale books may be purchased for business or promotional use or for special sales. For information, please write to:

Special Markets Department, Rodale Inc., 733 Third Avenue, New York, NY 10017

Men's Health is a registered trademark of Rodale Inc.

Printed in the United States of America

Rodale Inc. makes every effort to use acid-free ♾, recycled paper ♻.

Book design by the *Men's Health* and *Women's Health* Branded Books Design team: Mark Michaelson, Elizabeth Neal, Laura White, and Mike Smith, with George Karabotsos

Interior photos by Mitch Mandell
Hair and makeup by Colleen Kobrick

Cover design by Joe Heroun / Cover photo by Beth Bischoff

Library of Congress Cataloging-in-Publication Data is on file with the publisher.

ISBN-13: 978-1-60529-137-6

2 4 6 8 10 9 7 5 3   hardcover

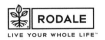

LIVE YOUR WHOLE LIFE™

We inspire and enable people to improve their lives and the world around them.

For Jennifer

CONTENTS

THE EASY WAY TO A HARD BODY

WIN THE WAR ON FAT
It's time to take control and transform your life with the *Men's Health* Diet.

HOW FIT ARE YOU?
Take the *Men's Health* Fitness Assessment and discover where your strengths and weaknesses lie.

THE MALE BODY AT 20, 30, 40, AND BEYOND!
Everything you need to know about your body—right now and for the future.

ANATOMY OF A POTBELLY
(And five reasons you might still be fat.)

WHY THE SMARTEST DIET IS NO DIET AT ALL
How to turn fat into muscle without giving up anything, ever (seriously).

HOW TO TRICK YOUR BODY INTO BURNING FAT
Meet your body's best defense against weight gain: more muscle.

THE *MEN'S HEALTH* RULES OF THE RIPPED!
Seven simple rules that will set you up for a lifetime of looking great.

FOREWORD

I lost my gut for America's glory.

True story. As a teen, I was overweight, and it took a stint in the Navy to whip me into shape—and a career at *Men's Health* to keep me in fighting trim.

But how did I get that gut in the first place? Like a lot of people, I nurtured it into being as I grew up. My mom was out working afternoons, so there was nobody around to bug me once I stepped off the school bus. I'd return home, plop down in the kitchen, and eat. Sometimes I would chow on tasty snacks I'd drag home from fast-food land. Sometimes I'd binge on whatever cookies, chips, or candy my older brother, Eric, might have missed. He obviously wasn't very attentive, because there was plenty for me to eat. And eat. And eat.

It got to the point where my brother would come around with his friends, point at me, and snicker, "Watch the big animal. It's feeding."

Thanks, bro. By poking me in my burgeoning belly, you were doing me a favor, I know.

Since then, I've learned a ton about physiology, nutrition, exercise science, and health. My career as a health journalist demanded it. But as I pored over the scientific journals and fought my way through the charts and tables, I've been motivated by the same biology lesson I learned back in the Navy: survival of the fittest.

No, not mere survival of the fittest. It goes way beyond that. It's the *happiness* of the fittest. The *sexiness* of the fittest. The *healthfulness* of the fittest. The *self-confidence* of the fittest. The *ka-ching* of the fittest. The connections between weight and life rewards are amply proven in the scientific literature. Lots of people, from romantic partners to business partners, take clues about your fitness to lead, your fitness to love, and your fitness to stick around from the overall state of your physical fitness.

That's right— vanity rules.

I won't comment about whether that's good or bad, but we all know that the health bias exists. It's an advantage you shouldn't cast aside carelessly. Every word we publish in *Men's Health* magazine serves that larger purpose: to help our readers seize the maximum advantage in health, fitness, and sex, and to succeed in life. And that that advantage begins with how much you weigh.

Weight is fate, my friends.

So when my colleague Steve Perrine proposed writing The *Men's Health* Diet, to distill the wisdom of 20 years of publishing into one slim (slimming) volume, it had a certain ring of familiarity. It was almost like the snide challenge my brother threw down to me as a teenager, minus the snide part. Can we help our readers rise to the occasion, and conquer the big animal that's lurking within, and spilling out over a stressed beltline?

Of course we can.

After all, *Men's Health* has helped tens of millions of men around the world—32 editions and counting—to conquer difficulties with their own equators. Why couldn't we put that advantage between two book covers, and help even more?

You're holding the results of that quest in your hands. Steve Perrine knows more about losing weight than practically anybody on the planet, steeped as he is in the *Men's Health* way. And now you can benefit from the best of weight-loss theory and practice from these pages. The lean belly you've always wanted is here. Maybe the six-pack, too.

And no need to endure snide comments from my brother, Eric, to get there.

Here's to the new you.

We've been expecting you.

David Zinczenko
EDITOR-IN-CHIEF
Men's Health magazine

ACKNOWLEDGMENTS

One summer's day in 1991, while taking out the recycling, I glanced down at the newspaper and saw an advertisement for a junior-level job at a new magazine called *Men's Health*. I drove my family out to Emmaus, Pennsylvania, to apply.

I didn't get that job.

Luckily, another position opened up soon after, and from that moment on, I've been fortunate to work with the greatest team of journalists, publishers, and health-care professionals ever assembled. In particular:

Maria Rodale and the Rodale family, who have been fighting to awaken us to the connection between our health and our environment for more than 60 years. I hope this book brings readers one step closer to realizing a healthier future.

David Zinczenko, whose support, encouragement, and grace under pressure have made possible my endeavors and those of many others at Rodale Inc.

My brilliant co-authors, Adam Bornstein and Heather Hurlock.

George Karabotsos, Debbie McHugh, Laura White, Mark Michaelson, Mike Smith, Theresa Dougherty, Ruth Davis Konigsberg, and the team at *Men's Health* Books.

The editors of *Men's Health* and *Women's Health* magazines, especially Adam Campbell, for his exercise expertise; Clint Carter, for his nutritional insights; Bill Phillips and Steve Borkowski for their Web and marketing support; and Peter Moore, for his inspiring calm and professionalism.

The staff of *Best Life* magazine.

Karen Rinaldi, Chris Krogermeier, Beth Lamb, Erin Williams, and the team at Rodale Books.

Fotoulla Euripidou, Meridith Lampert, and Philavong Chanda for their dedication to getting just the facts, ma'am. Lisa Krueger, Allison Falkenberry, Agnes Hansdorfer, Brett LeVecchio, Erin Clinton, and Allison Keane, who have helped us to spread the word about *The Men's Health Diet*.

The late Elaine Kaufman, for her heaping plates of wisdom and encouragement.

And my daughters Dominique, Anaïs, and Zoë, without whom I would have a lot more money—and a lot less joy.

INTRODUCTION
THE EASY WAY TO A HARD BODY

Inside your body, at this very moment, a war is raging.

On one side, the good guy: Muscle. Muscle is like the doorman of your own personal nightclub. It's his job to make you look good, attracting the cute girls and keeping out the riffraff.

The riffraff, in this case, is a guy called Fat.

Fat hates Muscle, and the feeling is mutual. Fat wants to fill your nightclub with all his fat, lazy friends, who will just sit around bumming free drinks, eating all the peanuts at the bar, and scaring away the women.

And Fat wants to run Muscle out of town.

You know which side you're rooting for. Muscle literally burns fat for energy, which is why building and maintaining muscle is the key to losing flab and sculpting the lean, toned body you've always wanted. Muscle will boost your metabolism, helping you to burn calories day and night. Muscle will heighten your testosterone level, keeping aging at bay and your sex drive revving. Muscle will help protect you from everything from heart disease to back pain, from arthritis to depression, all while garnering you more attention from women and potential employers—and less attention from doctors and collection agencies.

But here's the problem: In this war, Fat will always have an unfair advantage. The only way Muscle can win is with your help.

The Men's Health Diet will show you how to win that battle. It will help you build muscle and burn away fat while eating the very best foods on the planet and never, ever feeling hungry. It will make you stronger, leaner, and healthier than you've ever been before. It will help you to look, feel, and live better than ever. And it will start to take effect, well, pretty much from your very first bite.

This is the plan that will help you turn Fat into Muscle, once and for all.

Ready to dig in?

A BETTER YOU, FAST

The Men's Health Diet is a complete nutrition and fitness plan designed to transform your body quickly and easily—or, more accurately, to help your body transform itself. (Hey, why should you do all the work?) It's a complete mind/body plan that will take you exactly where you want to go: to the very best point in your life. The point at which you are the healthiest, fittest, and happiest you've ever been. And it's designed to keep you there for decades to come.

And here's the crazy part: It's not hard at all. All you need are a few simple secrets. And you're holding those secrets in your hands right now.

HOT TIPS

10 TIPS THAT CAN CHANGE YOUR LIFE IN 10 SECONDS OR LESS

1 Drink your milk. Think you're getting a nutritional boost from your morning cereal? Up to 40 percent of the vitamins in fortified cereals dissolve in the milk. If you don't drink the leftover cow juice, you're not getting the fancy-pants nutrients!

2 Ice it, ace it. Drink ice-cold water before and during exercise. Studies show that the cold stuff can improve endurance by about 23 percent. And ice water forces your body to expend calories warming it up, boosting your metabolism as well.

3 Lift, damn it! Expressing emotion while lifting increases muscle strength by up to 25 percent. (Of course, it also increases your risk of being tossed out of the gym by the same percentage . . .) Or get someone to scream at you: You'll be able to lift 5 to 8 percent more weight if you get encouragement from a trainer or workout partner.

4 Bribe yourself fit. Bet a colleague (like that guy who's not so secretly gunning for your job) 50 bucks that you can stick to your workout program for 6 months. Studies show that those who do achieve an average 97 percent success rate. Alternate plan? Schedule your workouts, then put $5 in a jar for each one you make. Pledge the money toward something sweet, like new golf clubs or a trip to Vegas.

5 Pick the red one. Red cabbage has 15 times as much wrinkle-fighting beta-carotene as green cabbage. Red bell peppers have up to nine times as much vitamin C as green ones.

6 Spear a hangover. To reduce the severity of a hangover, order a side of asparagus. When South Korean researchers exposed a group of human liver cells to asparagus extract, the extract suppressed free radicals and more than doubled the effects of two enzymes responsible for metabolizing alcohol.

7 Listen to your feet. If you can hear yourself running, you're setting yourself up for injury. That pounding comes from bad form, and it means you're risking harm to your joints. Keep your feet close to the ground and use a quick, shuffling stride.

8 Don't buy wheat bread. Huh? Isn't it good for me? Actually, "wheat bread" is often just white bread dyed with molasses to make it look dark. Look instead for "100 percent whole wheat" or "whole grain." Even better: rye bread. Swedish researchers found that 8 hours after people ate rye, they felt less hungry than those who noshed wheat bread, thanks to rye's high fiber content.

9 Cheat with a dumbbell. Lift a dumbbell weight as many times as you can. Then, when you can't complete one more repetition, use your free hand to help push your weighted hand through another rep. Once you're at the top of the move, remove your free hand and slowly lower the weight. Studies show that negative resistance exercises like this are more effective at muscle building than standard exercises.

10 Dry off head to toe. Literally. After a shower, you'll prevent a chill by drying your head and neck first. But more important, you'll also reduce the risk of anything nasty from the shower floor making its way up your body.

As you've walked through life, you've no doubt noticed that some guys just seem to look and feel their best all the time. Their bodies are fit, their clothes are pressed, and their shoes are as shiny and clean as Jennifer Aniston's cheekbones. Whether through luck or skill or inheritances of sweet genes and hefty bank accounts, they've got it made. These guys tend to show up in the expected places: the Super Bowl, the Olympics, the Fortune 500, *Ocean's Eleven*, and Lady Gaga's vacation videos.

HOT TIP #11

Get steely, Dan.
Steel-cut oats trigger twice as many immunity-boosting white blood cells as rolled, quick-cooking oats. Sure, they take up more time, but so do sick days.

But these guys are the exceptions. Most of us won't be starring alongside Drew Brees, George Clooney, or Kobe Bryant anytime soon. We don't have rich uncles, personal trainers, executive chefs, or multimillion-dollar endorsement deals. Most of us are just, well, regular guys: We work hard, we play hard, and we're pretty damn good at what we do. But we're also balancing about a million and one daily dramas, demands, and drudgeries, trying to figure out the right path forward as we're bombarded from all sides by health and nutrition choices that are as twisted and tangled as a Goldman Sachs balance sheet.

Any regular guy who wants to be better than he is right now, physically and mentally, needs a leg up—a little advice he can trust, a big brother who's been around the block and can help him navigate the Sudoku puzzle of life.

That's why I've created *The Men's Health Diet*. For the last quarter century, men who want to improve their bodies and their lives have been turning to *Men's Health* as the ultimate source of fitness, nutrition, and weight-loss information anywhere in the world. From its first issue in 1987 to the international powerhouse that it is today, *Men's Health* has collected, analyzed, studied, and refined the most authoritative research ever conducted on sculpting and enhancing the male body into its fittest, healthiest form. And every bit of advice we proffer is vetted—by the latest science, by the top experts, and by our own independent testing—to ensure that it works.

At the Energy Center, our on-site fitness facility, we try out the latest exercise gear, techniques, and strategies. In our library, which is the largest private medical library in the world, we keep a database that tracks and sorts every study published in every top scientific journal in the world. At the Rodale Institute—the 333-acre experimental farm operated by our parent company, Rodale Inc.— we unearth the healthiest foods on the planet and discover the best ways to raise, harvest, and consume them. And in our test kitchens and company cafeterias, we cook up and taste-test those foods, using recipes we've honed over years of nutritional research.

Along the way, we've discovered that fitness and nutrition are at the core of just about every area a man can hope to improve on in his life, from looking great (both men and women rate fit guys as up to 43 percent more attractive) to gaining financial footing (one study at New York University found that people who carry an extra 40 pounds make 20 percent less than their slimmer colleagues) to improving his whole outlook on life (nutrients like folate and omega-3 fatty acids, which you'll read more about in Chapters 6 and 7, have been shown to boost intelligence, mood, and even sexual function).

> **HOT TIP #12**
>
> **Don't skip out.**
> There is a 61 percent likelihood that after missing one workout you'll also skip an exercise session the following week, according to a UK study. Keep that in mind the next time you consider forgoing a trip to the gym.

And along the way, we've tapped every expert source of information for an answer for every conundrum facing the modern man, from how to get a closer shave (do it after you shower, so the steam has time to soften your beard) to how to get a better abs workout (you can do 17 percent more situps if you're properly hydrated, studies show) to how to trick yourself into eating less (scientists at the University of Massachusetts found that people who turn off the TV before eating consume an average of 288 fewer calories). With that kind of positive, practical, life-altering information, one humble magazine has grown into a powerhouse with 38 international editions, 20 million readers worldwide, and more than 85 million page views every month on its Web site. It's also the kind of authoritative research that has gone into designing the Rules of the Ripped—the backbone of the *Men's Health* Diet—and informs the 101 life-altering tips you'll find sprinkled throughout these pages.

HOT TIP #13

Don't do drive-through. USDA scientists recently found that men eat 500 more calories on days they consume fast foods compared with days they don't. Junk begets junk....

So that's why you can trust me when I say that the distance between where you are now and where you want to be is smaller than you think.

AN EXTRAORDINARY PLAN FOR REGULAR GUYS

Think about this: According to a University of Connecticut study, men add a pound of fat a year from the ages of 25 to 45. That's hardly any at all from one year to the next, but over the course of several years, it explains a lot—and it seems like an inevitable, unstoppable march, especially once you're halfway down that path. But reversing that course doesn't require as dramatic a life change as you might think. When USDA scientists studied the eating habits of 8,837 adults, they found that on a typical day, overweight adults eat a mere 100 calories more than their normal-weight peers—the equivalent of having a cookie with your 3 p.m. coffee.

A hundred calories? Come on! Really? If that's true, then why does it seem so hard for most of us to get the bodies we want? Why do we feel miles away from the Pitts, Damons, and Mannings of the world? Because we're surrounded by a world of bad: bad advice, bad choices, and above all, bad food. (And that includes plenty of stuff being marketed as "health food.") The fact is, trusting food manufacturers to watch over your body is like trusting Michael Vick to house-sit your dog. Thanks to our nutritionally bankrupt food supply, more than 7 out of every 10 guys you went to high school with are overweight or obese (if

> **HOT TIP #14**
>
> **Go dark.** In almost every case, the darker the color of a bean or vegetable, the more nutrients it contains. Black beans beat navy beans and broccoli tops cauliflower, every time.

they weren't already that way when you were sitting next to them in algebra; the percentage of kids ages 12 to 19 who are overweight or obese nearly quadrupled between the mid-'70s and the mid-2000s). How did this happen?

It wasn't some tsunami of fat that washed over us all. It was a mere 100 calories a day. Today and yesterday and the day before that . . .

Well, guess what? Tomorrow is a brand-new day.

REBUILDING A BETTER YOU

If you've tried diet-and-fitness plans before, you've probably discovered one serious problem with most of them: They're about sacrificing, about cutting down, about giving up.

Guys hate that.

But the *Men's Health* Diet is different, in several ways:

• **IT'S ABOUT LIVING YOUR BEST LIFE.** One of the coolest aspects of the *Men's Health* Diet is that you can pretty much cheat any time you want—as long as you're cheating with the best. Ice cream? Sure. Pork chops? Okay. Greasy delivery pizza? Yes, actually. You can indulge your taste buds any time you want, but with one small caveat: You're only allowed to indulge in the best. That means the best-tasting, healthiest, smartest versions of your favorite foods—even foods that come at you through your car window. (The 250 Best Foods for Men—from pepperoni slices to french fries—can be found in Chapter 10.) Once you discover that you can still order a fast-food burger but save 800 flab-inducing calories and boost your muscle-building protein intake simply by choosing the best of the best, you'll see how very easy this diet plan is!

HOT TIP #15

Cut the paper. In a Cornell study, people who ate from paper plates with plastic utensils tended to consider their food just a snack, while those who ate the same food off "real" plates considered their food a meal. Result: Those who eat off paper plates are more likely to seek out food later.

• **IT'S ABOUT WORKING WITH YOUR BODY, NOT AGAINST IT.** The groundbreaking science that's emerged in just the past year has shown that when it comes to guys and food, timing is everything. In fact, your body goes through periods every day when it wants to burn fat, build muscle, and grow leaner and stronger. It just needs the right fuel at the right time. (That's why we'll have you eating the majority of your calories in the first half of the day.) Simply by knowing how to time your meals, you'll prime your body for maximum muscle and superfast weight loss.

• **IT'S ABOUT EATING MORE, NOT LESS.** We mean more good food, the kind of stuff your body craves. In fact, eating as much food as your body needs will actually be a challenge: Food is the fuel that will burn away fat and build lean, strong muscle. That's the philosophy behind what we call the *Men's Health* Nutrition System, and you'll learn all about it in the coming pages.

• **IT'S ABOUT GROWING BIGGER AND STRONGER.** Too many diets are about downsizing your body. But the *Men's Health* Diet is about upgrading. In an upcoming chapter, you'll learn more about that war that's raging inside your body, the war between fat and muscle. Who wins that war will determine not just what your body will look like, but how well and how long it will continue to function. (Get ready to muster the troops!)

> **HOT TIP #16**
>
> **Bone up.** Research suggests that omega-3s in salmon can boost bone density. Next time you barbecue, switch beef burgers for salmon patties.

• **IT'S ABOUT HAVING FUN.** The *Men's Health* Muscle System (see Chapter 8) is a fitness plan that's not based on sweat and sacrifice. In fact, it actually requires you to enjoy yourself. Sure, there's some work involved, but once you understand the physiological principles of stress management and active rest—whether that means shooting hoops, playing tag, hitting the slopes, or chasing the elusive rainbow trout—you'll see just how critical having fun is to reaching your fitness goals.

GET READY TO CHANGE YOUR LIFE!

As a *Men's Health* editor for nearly 20 years, I've been lucky to be part of the best health and fitness editorial team ever assembled. But I'm also something else: a classic *Men's Health* success story.

I joined the team back in the early 1990s, when the magazine was just getting off the ground. Like a lot of folks in the publishing industry, I was pretty skeptical about the idea of a "men's health magazine." Health, fitness, and nutrition weren't the kinds of things "real" men talked about. Sports, politics, women, and the stock market—that was the stuff of male conversation. And if your pants grew tighter than Nicole Kidman's forehead and your back felt like a dozen stilettoed divorce attorneys were taking a hike up your vertebrae? Well, that is just the way it was. If you wanted to lose weight or feel healthier, then you took up "jogging" or you followed the latest diet trend—secretly. And sometimes, it even worked.

But not often, and not for long.

That's about where I was back in the early 1990s. Like a lot of people, I was eating low-fat and fighting energy shortages by "carbo-loading." Big day tomorrow? A huge plate of pasta (no olive oil, please!) was just the ticket to keep sharp. That 3 p.m. slump? I'd often wander down to the deli and help myself to not one but two bagels—hey, no fat, no problem, right? (Little did I know that I was helping myself to nearly 600 extra calories a day!) By the time I was 27 years old, I was upgrading (or downgrading, if you will) to size 36 jeans—5 inches more than I had sported freshman year of college.

Indeed, last summer, while I was packing up my oldest daughter for her own freshman year of college, I came across a photo of her that was taken on her first day of kindergarten. And my first reaction was "Why is she standing there with Michael Moore?"

> **HOT TIP #17**
>
> **Go nuts to stay sane.** A study in the *Journal of the American Medical Association* found that those men who consumed the most vitamin E—from food sources, not supplements—had a 67 percent lower risk for Alzheimer's disease than those eating the least.

And my second reaction was "Holy jiggling juggernauts of Jell-O! That's me!"

But that's not me any longer. Today, thanks to following the fitness, nutrition, and stress-management advice we publish every month, my body looks a lot more like it did at 17 than at 27. (And yeah, that means size 31 jeans, even at age 46.) *Men's Health* has literally changed my life. And it's changed the lives of tens of thousands of other men as well.

Now it's your turn.

In this war, Fat will always have an unfair advantage. The only way Muscle can win is with your help. The *Men's Health* Diet will show you how to win that battle.

JUMPSTART
A QUICK LOOK AT THE PRINCIPLES OF *THE MEN'S HEALTH DIET*

HOW TO GET FAST & LEAN:
THE *MEN'S HEALTH* NUTRITION SYSTEM

WHAT TO EAT *The Men's Health Diet* is based on eight superfood groups, foods scientifically proven to get you lean, fast. In fact, all you need to remember is:

Fiber-rich grains
Avocados, oils, and healthy fats
Spinach and leafy greens
Turkey and lean meats

Legumes
Eggs and dairy
Apples and other fruits
Nuts and seeds

 + High-quality protein, mood-boosting folate, brain-building omega-3s, and fiber-rich carbs like whole fruits and vegetables

— Refined carbs, salt, high-fructose corn syrup and other sweeteners, and trans fats

HOW MUCH TO EAT Instead of counting calories or obsessing over portion sizes, pack your plate with nutrient-dense, fiber-rich foods; pay attention to your body's signals; and only eat until you're full. General portion guidelines can be found in the palm of your hand. Literally:

MEATS: The size of your palm
VEGETABLES AND FRUITS: As big as a tight fist
OILS AND OTHER HEALTHY FATS: A teaspoon is equal to the end of your

thumb, from the knuckle up
LEGUMES: Whatever fits in the palm of your hand
GRAINS: The size of a tight fist
DAIRY: The size of your palm

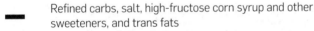

5 MEALS	CALORIES PER MEAL			+ BEVERAGES/DESSERT	200
	BREAKFAST	**SNACK**	**LUNCH**	**SNACK**	**DINNER**
	500 to 750	200 to 300	400 to 500	200 to 300	500 to 600

The Men's Health Diet is all about eating more food, not less. By following our Rules of the Ripped, you will fill your body with the nutrients you need to stoke your metabolism, blast belly fat, and build lean, long-lasting muscle. Here's a quick overview of what you'll be eating each day:

THE *MEN'S HEALTH* MUSCLE SYSTEM

The *Men's Health* Muscle System will turbocharge your weight loss and help you pack on lean, powerful muscle. It is a revolutionary new workout prescription based on time—not on boring sets and reps. You'll move quickly from one resistance exercise to the next, doing as many reps as you can in 30 seconds, then resting for 15 seconds before moving on to the next exercise.

WEIGHT WORKOUTS PER WEEK **3**

DURATION OF WORKOUTS IN MINUTES **30**

ADDITIONAL FAT-BURNING ACTIVITIES: Choose from a variety of fun activities, from hiking to golf to playing tag with the neighborhood kids. A weekly session of "having fun" is a mandatory part of your new workout plan!

THE *MEN'S HEALTH* RULES OF THE RIPPED

RULE 1: "I Will Eat Protein with Every Meal and Every Snack." (Eat 10 to 15 grams per snack, 30 per meal.)

RULE 2: "I Will Never Eat the World's Worst Breakfast." (The worst breakfast is no breakfast at all.)

RULE 3: "I Will Eat Before and After Exercise." (Eat a mix of protein and carbs.)

RULE 4: "I Will Eat It if It Grows on a Tree" (Add as many fruits, vegetables, nuts, and beans to your diet as you can stomach.)

RULE 5: "I Will Eat the Salad, Even if It Makes Me Feel Girly." (Eat them in addition to your meals, not in place of them!)

RULE 6: "I Will Not Drink Sugar Water." (Watch your beverage calories.)

RULE 7: "I Will Stick to My Rules ~~100 Percent~~ 80 Percent of the Time." (Cheat whenever you want! We'll show you how.)

1

WIN THE WAR ON FAT

IT'S TIME TO TAKE CONTROL AND TRANSFORM YOUR LIFE WITH *THE MEN'S HEALTH DIET.*

If you're like most men, you've struggled to control your weight and keep the lean, defined musculature you remember from boyhood. Well, those days of struggle are over. If you want to turn fat into muscle and get into the best shape of your life, *The Men's Health Diet* will help you reach your goals. Your body is an amazing machine; get ready to fire it up!

And the first and easiest step toward achieving the body you've always wanted starts with changing the way you eat.

Malcolm Aylward, who lost 17 pounds on the *Men's Health* Diet in just 6 weeks and toned up his entire body, summed it up the best: "If you want to increase your fitness levels, your diet is 80 percent of the work. You can work out all you want, but if you're not eating well, you're not going to get the results."

And he's right. According to a 2010 study in the *Journal of the American Medical Association,* a whopping 72 percent of American men are either overweight or obese.

HOT TIP #18

Find the right chemistry. Men with high levels of bisphenol-A (BPA) in their bloodstreams are 2 to 4 times more likely to have problems with sperm quality. To cut BPA levels, reduce the amount of canned food you eat, and don't drink from or store food in plastics with a #7 at the bottom.

Our obesity epidemic poses a massive threat to public health. According to the National Institutes of Health, the health care costs associated with obesity are expected to double every decade. And it's not solely an American problem: According to some estimates, by the year 2030, nearly 2 billion people around the globe will be overweight or obese.

Now you may be thinking: "So all I need to do is lay off the Snickers bars and start running more, right?" Not quite. Weight-loss gurus will tell you that it's all a matter of willpower and that you need to drastically overhaul your life in order to get fit. But that's just not the truth. The reality is that most diet and exercise plans are designed to work in the short term and usually fail in the long run. (And if the plan fails? It must be your fault, because you didn't have the willpower to stick to it.)

Well, that's all bull. *The Men's Health Diet* has been designed to change this picture and to help you transform your body into what

He lost 11 pounds in 6 weeks!

SUCCESS *stories*

"I powered through each day."

TERRY WADSWORTH, 61, Edgewater, FL

STARTING WEIGHT 220 LBS / **WEIGHT AFTER 6 WEEKS 209 LBS** / **HEIGHT 6'0"**

The last 10 pounds are always the hardest to lose. But that was Terry Wadsworth's goal when he started the *Men's Health* Diet. And in the end, he was able to surpass that, plus achieve a leaner, healthier body overall.

Discovering a New Way of Eating

Terry decided to try *the Men's Health* Diet because he wanted eating habits that would fit his lifestyle. But he had initial reservations about parts of the plan: "Eating both before and after my workout was something that I didn't normally do in the past, and it took some effort to make it part of my routine," he said. But he soon discovered that the "guidelines made perfect sense and were easy to follow."

Powering through the Day

One unexpected benefit was a change in Terry's mood. Not only did he feel more upbeat, but he also noticed that his energy levels were up and remained more consistent throughout the day. "Putting a big emphasis on breakfast really made a difference for me," he said. "It powered me through the day." He added that the good feeling he got from being on the diet, along with his steady weight loss, helped him stay motivated to continue with the plan.

Getting a Leaner Payoff

As his time on The *Men's Health* Diet progressed, Terry saw his body slim and his clothes fit. And he wasn't the only one who noticed the change. "I was asked by my family and friends alike what I was doing," he said. Terry had always wanted to be "lean, athletic, and healthy. The *Men's Health* Diet got me to those goals without imposing overly restrictive lifestyle changes. It seems natural."

3

it should be—a muscle-building, fat-burning machine. In just 6 weeks, you could lose up to 15 pounds—or more!—while building muscle and sculpting your dream body. To initiate this change, you won't need to drastically overhaul your life. That's because the *Men's Health* Diet has been designed with you in mind—your body, your schedule, your time. The main components of the plan are seven simple-to-follow rules—we call them the Rules of the Ripped. They're seven easy principles to follow that will keep you making the right food choices for your body, without having to make serious sacrifices. (Rule #2: "I will never eat the world's worst breakfast." That's all you need to do to start reshaping your body.) When you follow the Rules of the Ripped, weight loss isn't just easy—it's automatic! Plus, you'll build your meals around the *Men's Health* Nutrition System—a group of eight super-healthy superfoods that will speed weight loss, build energy, and even boost your mood. (You'll know these foods by the simple acronymn FAST & LEAN—learn more about them in Chapter 7!) And just to make things even easier, we've included recipes for terrific new fat-burning foods, and a list of the 250 Best Foods for Men. Sample any of them at any time, and watch the pounds disappear! More and more Americans are discovering that it really works.

> **HOT TIP #19**
>
> **Go nuts to stay sane.** A study in the Journal of the American Medical Association found that those men who consumed the most vitamin E—from food sources, not supplements—had a 67 percent lower risk for Alzheimer's disease than those eating the least.

Let's return to the story of Malcolm Aylward. At age 48, he was packing 245 pounds on his 6-foot-1 frame. He'd spent his whole life trying to get rid of those unwanted pounds, never with much success. But then he discovered the *Men's Health* Diet, and everything changed.

Malcolm reversed his diabetes in 6 weeks!

"I feel stronger, more athletic."

MALCOLM AYLWARD, 48, Machesney Park, IL

STARTING WEIGHT **245 LBS** / WEIGHT AFTER 6 WEEKS **228 LBS** / HEIGHT **6'1"**

Malcolm Aylward discovered the *Men's Health* Diet on menshealth.com after being inspired by watching the television show *Spartacus: Blood and Sand*. "I thought, if those actors can get whipped into shape for their roles, there's no reason I can't do it myself," he said.

Getting Hollywood Fit

Malcolm began the *Men's Health* Diet in conjunction with the *Men's Health* Muscle System. Once too tired to do anything after work, he now had the energy in the evening to complete his workouts.

"I feel stronger, more athletic," he said. "Everyday tasks, like mowing the lawn, are easier because I am more fit." His family and friends noticed the changes in his physical appearance and his mood, too. They told him he looked younger, stronger, more fit, and less stressed.

Unexpected Benefits

Malcolm had been diagnosed with type 2 diabetes and was having trouble controlling his blood sugar. But once he tried the *Men's Health* Diet, those troubles disappeared. The eating plan easily fit into his diabetic treatment, which recommended that he divide his meals into five small courses throughout the day to keep glucose levels even. Malcolm was even able to reverse his diabetes diagnosis!

Achieving a Lifelong Goal

With the help of the *Men's Health* Diet, Malcolm did something that he always hoped to do but was never able to accomplish—lose weight. "I figured it was time for a change," he said. Time to achieve the body I'd always wanted. And I'm getting there. I have to keep going. I'm not there yet, but already I am light-years away from where I was."

Malcolm had tried other diets before, but most of them—low-fat, low carb, low anything—required him to practice some kind of restrictive eating. And while he found that he lost weight using these plans, they left him feeling pretty bad. "I would always have an upset stomach, and I felt like I had no strength, no energy," he said. What's more, having been previously diagnosed with type 2 diabetes, Malcolm found that his eating habits weren't doing a very good job of helping him control his blood sugar and other diabetes symptoms.

But on the *Men's Health* Diet, Malcolm saw his blood sugar drop to normal levels as his pants size decreased. By combining the *Men's Health* Nutrition System with regular workouts, he saw his body become stronger and more athletic. His friends and family members told him that he looked younger and more fit. He found himself feeling less stressed and approaching each day with more energy than ever before. And he actually reversed his diabetes—something that a high-protein diet combined with resistance training has been proven to do, according to a 2010 study in Diabetes Care.

Is it possible that one plan can help you create a total mind and body change? Absolutely. And what incredible effects you'll see. Here's just a short list of the many ways *The Men's Health Diet* will change your life.

HOT TIP #20

Romp rigorously. One vigorous go-around in the bedroom blasts about 200 calories and doubles your heart rate. Twice a week? Shed nearly 6 pounds a year.

You'll Eat More Than Ever—And Never Feel Hungry

Here's a fact about most diets: They set you up for failure. If you've ever tried a restrictive diet program before, you know what I'm talking about. These plans are focused on "good" foods and "bad" foods, extensive calorie counting, or cutting entire food groups out

He lost 11 pounds in 6 weeks!

"I saved time—and saw better results."

PEISHU LI, 48, Plano, TX

STARTING WEIGHT **170 LBS** / WEIGHT AFTER 6 WEEKS **158 LBS** / HEIGHT **5'10"**

Peishu Li started the *Men's Health* Diet with the goal of reaching 160 pounds or less—but he was also looking for a way to stay healthy and eat well. He found all three.

Finding a Flexible Plan

Peishu had already been preparing his own food and eating multiple small meals throughout the day, so he found the "Rules of the Ripped"—the seven simple diet guidelines that define The *Men's Health* Diet—easy to incorporate into his schedule.

"Personally, I find strict formulas or counting calories just plain boring, inconvenient, and hard to stick to." Luckily, he found none of those elements on The *Men's Health* Diet.

Exercising as a Family Affair

Peishu's wife was so impressed by his weight loss that she decided to join him. "She started to do the circuit training with me," he said. "She loves the workout."

Peishu found that the *Men's Health* Muscle System helped him make his workouts more efficient. "It's actually saved my time, since I had been training about four times a week for about 60 minutes per session. The *Men's Health* Muscle System gave me better results, and I only had to work out three times a week; with 30 minutes per session," he said.

Making Changes for Life

In addition to beating his weight-loss goals, Peishu reaped other rewards from the *Men's Health* Diet. He's gotten leaner and stronger, and his muscles are now noticeably defined. He feels more energized throughout the day and has brought his previously elevated blood pressure levels back to normal. As a result, he plans to continue with what he's learned from the program.

"I've incorporated the *Men's Health* Diet into my long-term nutrition strategy and continue to live a healthy lifestyle," he said.

of your life. But you can only deprive your body of something for so long. Sooner or later, denying that craving for a slice of cheese pizza could lead you to the one moment when you break down and eat the entire pie. The good news is, there are no restrictions on the *Men's Health* Diet.

Instead, you'll be spreading out your eating over five meals and snacks made up of eight superfood groups, each designed to get you on the fast track to lean. In fact, that's what I've called them: FAST & LEAN superfoods. You'll read all about them in Chapter 7. With the right combination of whole foods, all chock-full of belly-filling fiber, protein, and other key nutrients, you'll end up eating more food but fewer calories, which is the perfect formula for weight-loss success.

> **HOT TIP #21**
>
> **Think before you eat.** British researchers found that people who reviewed their previous meals before chowing down ate 30 percent fewer calories than those who didn't. The theory: simply remembering what you've already eaten makes you less likely to overindulge.

It's a formula that's been proven time and again. A 2007 study in the *American Journal of Clinical Nutrition* compared weight loss in two groups. One group was instructed to eat a lot of whole foods (like those in the *Men's Health* Diet FAST & LEAN plan), while the other group was instructed to eat a low-fat diet. The whole-foods group ate 25 percent more food by volume and still lost an average of 5 pounds more. How? They were eating fewer calories, but they were still satisfied, thanks to the high nutrient and water content in the foods.

And that's what happens when you follow the *Men's Health* Diet, because you're replacing junk calories with nutritious calories. Indeed, a study in the *Journal of Food Composition and Analysis* determined that nearly one-third of the food most people eat is

He unveiled his six-pack!

SUCCESS *stories*

"I can look in the mirror and see abs!"

RICHARD CASADOS, 50, Albuquerque, NM

STARTING WEIGHT 142 LBS / **WEIGHT AFTER 6 WEEKS 136 LBS** / **HEIGHT 5'7"**

Richard Casados is a runner. He thought that his exercise routine was enough to keep his weight down and his body healthy, but he admits that his nutrition was not always the best. And although he was able to avoid becoming overweight, once he tried the *Men's Health* Diet, he was also able to transform his body into a much more defined and sculpted physique.

Balancing Diet and Exercise Lead to Big Results

Richard's most substantial payoff from the *Men's Health* Diet? Muscles. Although he had always worked out on a regular basis, the *Men's Health* Diet allowed him to incorporate strength training into his mostly cardio routine. He began by cutting down his running and biking schedule to 3 days each week, and adding in 3 days of weight lifting. He supplemented his workouts with the *Men's Health* Diet guidelines, which he found to be easy to follow.

By changing his eating habits and adding strength training to his routine, Richard lost weight but not muscle, which was just enough to drastically change his appearance.

"I feel much better physically, especially looking in the mirror and seeing abs and defined muscles," he said. "I was already thin, but having a six-pack and defined muscles makes me look like I did back when I was a US Army lean, mean, fighting machine."

It was the changes in his physical appearance, and his desire to lead a healthier life, that kept Richard motivated to keep up with the *Men's Health* Diet.

"If it is in you to want it," he said, "then you'll get it."

"Overall, I want to stay lean and fit by eating right and exercising with a combination of weight lifting and running or biking. I want to be able to compete in my age groups for years to come—at least up until 80."

9

pure junk. Five food types—sweets and desserts, soft drinks, fruit drinks, salty snacks, and alcohol—make up 30 percent of our calories. (Soda alone contributes more than 7 percent of the average person's daily calories!)

So your best weight-loss bet is not to eat less food, but to eat more. But it needs to be food that's high in nutrients and low in empty calories and fat-promoting ingredients. And on the *Men's Health* Diet you'll do just that. You'll be fueling your body with the finest foods out there. That means the best-tasting, healthiest, smartest versions of all of the foods you love—from take-out tacos to burgers hot off the grill. And when you need a break from the FAST & LEAN superfoods? Cheat at will—but do it with the very best cheat foods in the world, from fast-food burgers to delivery pizza. And I've done most of the hard work for you. With my list of the 250 Best Foods for Men (you'll find it in Chapter 10), you'll be able to customize this plan to fit your tastes, your goals, and your life!

> **HOT TIP #22**
>
> **Don't crowd your chow.** When picking food from a buffet, leave spaces between the foods you select. You could consume up to 20 percent fewer calories than if you pack your plate.

You'll Lose Fat—And Build Muscle!

Too many diet plans restrict calories, which is a really great way to lose weight in the short run—and gain it all back, and more, in the long run.

You've heard the term "yo-yo dieting" before, but you probably don't know what triggers the yo-yo effect. Blame it on evolution. When ancient man had trouble finding food—because of a prolonged drought, an ice age, or maybe a shortage of bows and arrows at the Neanderthal Cabela's—his body needed to be able to weather the hard times by using its store of body mass to keep its

He lost 12 pounds in 6 weeks!

SUCCESS *stories*

"I enjoy eating and didn't feel deprived of anything"

DAVID KROUSE, 37, Fruita, CA

STARTING WEIGHT 187 LBS / WEIGHT AFTER 6 WEEKS **175 LBS** / HEIGHT **5'10"**

The thought of baring your body in public is often a good motivator to get in shape. It was this thought—and an impending beach trip to Mexico—that drew David Krouse to try the *Men's Health* Diet. He'd tried other diets before, but this program seemed to him the most realistic and easy to follow, and was perfect for shaping up with a deadline in mind.

Finding a Trusted Plan

David was attracted to the stability of the *Men's Health* Diet plan. "I trust the advice given by *Men's Health*," he said. He was further enticed by the program's simplicity as well as the variety of food options offered and helpful guidelines and tips given.

"I particularly liked the specificity, as I am not a really creative kind of person and I like having clear advice and direction," he said.

He added that while on the *Men's Health* Diet, "I felt good. It wasn't drastically different from what I had been doing, but it was good to have some structure. I never felt starved or anything. I had plenty of energy for my workouts. I really enjoy eating, and I didn't really feel deprived of anything."

Staying Lean after the Vacation

Although it was his trip to Mexico that kept David motivated throughout the 6-week plan, it was the lasting results that gave him the biggest reward. In the end, his efforts paid off. His sister told him his upper body muscles were looking "huge," his wife commented that he'd noticeably lost a lot of fat, and several of his co-workers said that he looked leaner.

"I don't have delusions of being a Brad Pitt or Hugh Jackman," he said, "but if I can improve my overall health, I'm happy. And if I look a little better along the way, all the better."

11

vital organs functioning. And guess what kind of tissue a hungry body burns first?

Muscle.

Here's why: Muscle burns a lot of calories—up to 6 a day per pound just by being there. Fat, on the other hand, burns a mere 2 or so calories a day. So if your body is in starvation mode and needs to lose weight, what weight will it want to drop? Right—muscle weight. Sure, when you restrict calories, you lose fat, but you lose muscle too. And with it, you lose muscle's fat-burning power. A study in the *Journal of Applied Physiology* found that calorie restriction (decreasing caloric intake by 16 to 20 percent) decreases bone mass, muscle mass, and strength.

> **HOT TIP #23**
>
> **Arm yourself.**
> Want bigger, stronger arms? Stop concentrating on your biceps. Triceps—the muscles on the back of your upper arm—make up 70 percent of your upper arm musculature. Focus on these to fill out your sleeves.

And that's exactly what happens when we follow a traditional diet plan. Once we stop "dieting," we go back to the same way of eating—but this time, without that valuable higher calorie burn we got from having more muscle. The more restrictive the diet, the more muscle you'll lose, and the more flab you'll regain over the long haul.

But the *Men's Health* Diet doesn't require you to starve yourself, cut out your favorite foods, or lose muscle. (And if you incorporate the *Men's Health* Muscle System into your weight-loss plan, you'll actually build muscle and burn even more calories!) Plus . . .

You'll Have More Energy—And See Results Faster!

Recent research suggests that when it comes to eating—and ultimately, to shedding fat and building muscle—when you eat is just as important as what you eat. On the *Men's Health* Diet, you'll be providing your body with the fuel it needs when it needs it the most: in the morning, and before and after you work out.

The results of one study reported that your risk of obesity increases 450 percent if you regularly skip breakfast. That's right, by 450 percent. But by consuming a protein-rich morning meal, you'll pull your body out of the fuel-deprived state it got into while you were sleeping and into the fat-burning, muscle-building zone. A 2008 study at Virginia Commonwealth University found that people who ate a large, protein-rich breakfast lost significantly more weight than those who consumed smaller morning meals with less protein. Unfortunately, our food industry has conditioned us to eat sugar-laden, refined carbs in the morning, which is the exact opposite of what our bodies need. *The Men's Health Diet* will show you how to fight back against crazy morning carbo-loading and get the protein you need to burn fat all day and all night.

You'll also be able to build even more muscle by scheduling your meals around your workouts. Dutch and British researchers reported that eating before training speeds muscle growth and helps your body increase strength and burn fat more effectively. Plus, independent studies by Finnish and British scientists discovered that, in addition to helping you build muscle faster, eating a healthy balance of protein and carbs both before and after exercising can speed your recovery time and help to reduce inflammation after a tough training session.

> **HOT TIP #24**
>
> **Embrace ginger spice.** Two grams of ground ginger a day can reduce soreness and help enhance new muscle growth, say researchers.

You'll Protect Your Body from Disease—Without Drugs!

Folate is crucial for proper brain and body functioning, according to Harvard researchers. Low levels of folate are linked to depression, reduced energy levels, and even memory loss. A study in the *American Journal of Clinical Nutrition* found that those with low folate levels have an increased risk of impaired cognitive function and dementia. A study in the journal Psychotherapy and Psychosomatics showed that low folate levels are found in depressed members of the general U.S. population. And it's not just your mind that suffers: Folate deficiency has been implicated in most of the major diseases of our time. It leads to an increased risk of obesity, stroke, heart disease, and even cancer.

HOT TIP #25

Bribe yourself slim. When a craving hits, bribe yourself thin. Instead of munching, put money into a box every time you want a snack. The growing pile of dough will be a reminder that you can overpower your urges. When you've saved enough cash, use it to splurge on a non-food reward.

You can reverse your risk for all these diseases and, within weeks, see noticeable improvements in your mood and brain function simply by following the guidelines of the *Men's Health* Diet. Studies show that adding folate-rich greens to your diet reduces fatigue, improves energy levels, and helps battle depression, something supplements can't do. In a review of studies in the *Journal of Psychopharmacology*, the authors concluded that depressed individuals should try increasing their folate levels in order to improve treatment outcomes.

By incorporating the *Men's Health* Diet guidelines into your daily schedule, you'll also increase your intake of omega-3 fatty acids—healthy fats that can cut your risk of everything from heart disease and stroke to arthritis and asthma. These nutrients are essential in boosting your mood and promoting brain health. Research suggests that people who eat the most omega-3-rich foods live longer and have less abdominal fat than those who eat less. And don't worry if you're not a seafood eater—omega-3s can be found in a multitude of other foods, from walnuts to kiwifruit.

Plus, not only are the FAST & LEAN foods healthier for you, they're tastier, too. Why? Because our taste buds evolved to crave flavor, and foods get their flavors from nutrients. The tartness of berries tells of their massive vitamin loads, the fat in fish delivers healthy omega-3s, and the bitterness of chocolate carries a dose of antioxidants.

You'll Rev Up Your Sex Life!

Men who are obese are five times as likely to suffer from erectile dysfunction (ED) than men who are of normal weight. To make things worse, a diet high in saturated and trans fats actually lowers your libido by decreasing testosterone levels. The foods on the *Men's Heath* Diet reverse this equation, slimming down your body and boosting your performance in bed.

Even those of us who don't need to lose pounds will see an improvement in lovemaking by using the *Men's Health* Muscle System. Good sex requires good cardiovascular and respiratory health: Research reported at the 2010 meeting of the American Urological Association showed that sexual function scores were highest in men who exercised. Here's why: Exercise boosts blood flow to all our organs, including the one between your legs. That means firmer erections that are less likely to flag when the going gets hot and heavy.

So there you have it. What's not to love about a plan that allows you to eat better versions of the foods you love while helping you become a stronger, healthier, happier version of yourself? It's time to get started! Your new body is waiting.

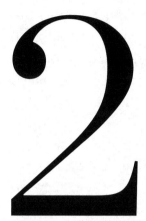

2

HOW FIT ARE YOU?
TAKE THE *MEN'S HEALTH* FITNESS ASSESSMENT AND DISCOVER WHERE YOUR STRENGTHS AND WEAKNESSES LIE.

Like most men, you've probably stepped out of the shower, caught a glimpse of yourself in the bathroom mirror, and thought, *Not so bad.* Stand up a little straighter, suck the gut in just a tad, and you're okay. Not that Matt Damon needs to be looking over his shoulder to see if you're going to take the Bourne series away from him, but as a torchbearer for the male gender, you'll do.

We all have ways of fooling ourselves into thinking we're fitter, stronger, healthier than we are. But in reality, no matter how hard we try to exercise and eat right, all of us are locked into repeated motions, positions, and habits that, day in and day out, take their toll on our bodies. Long days slumped in front of the computer, endless commutes nestled in the driver's seat—hours upon hours, for week after week, of your body doing things it just wasn't built to do. Over time, as you remain locked in bad postures, some muscles shorten and tighten, others stretch and weaken, and the natural alignment of your body gets tweaked and tweaked some more until it's totally out of whack. Even if you do get to the gym regularly, those workouts aren't necessarily fixing what's getting slowly, inexorably broken.

That's because almost everyone who hits the gym or works out at home is committing the cardinal sin of exercise: having poor form. Most people don't know how to perform the most basic exercises correctly, and the handful of training sessions you took when you signed up at the gym probably didn't arm you with all the tools you need to make a real difference. Poor exercise technique is the number-one reason many gym-goers struggle to make real, long-lasting changes to their bodies. According to military brass, 27 percent of young Americans are so out of shape they can't even serve our country. The only way to change that figure—whether your goal is to battle the Taliban or just the telltale signs of aging—is to exercise consistently. But you can't trade in your spare tire for a six-pack unless

> **HOT TIP #26**
>
> **Uncover the flax.**
> Sprinkle ground flaxseed over cereal, pancakes, yogurt, and smoothies. It's an easy way to add belly-filling fiber and omega-3 fatty acids. Not a fan of flax? Try pumpkin or sunflower seeds—two more great sources of healthy fats and some fiber.

you identify where you're weakest, choose the right exercises to counteract those weaknesses, and perform those exercises correctly, time after time.

That's what this book will help you do. Once you know how to identify these problem areas and improve how you move, you'll experience a better workout every time you exercise. And in no time, the words "struggle" and "plateau" will be a thing of the past.

HOT TIP #27

Keep your mouth busy. Chew gum while you prepare food or whenever you're surrounded by stuff you don't need to eat.

Think about it: When you perform an exercise incorrectly, or focus on one or two body parts at the expense of others, it sets your body up for a series of failures. One poor rep becomes 10. Multiply that by 3 sets performed 3 times per week, and that's 90 reps of joint-straining, imbalance-creating movements on your body. Continue multiplying and it becomes easy to see why you haven't experienced success, despite your best efforts. If you're doing the exercises wrong, or have a hidden weakness, not only will you see limited results, but you're also going to get hurt.

In fact, a 27-year review of gym injuries found that nearly 70 percent of all lifting injuries were either sprains, strains, or soft tissue injuries caused by poor form (only 0.2 percent were concussions, which means that no matter how poor your form, you're probably not going to be dropping weights on your head). And even if you're doing the exercises correctly, you might still be sending yourself to the couch. That's because researchers at Nova Southeastern University, in Florida, found that men who lift weights are more likely to have shoulder pain and other upper body injuries that restrict exercise than those who never lift weights. The reason: Poor training programs that overemphasize your chest and bicepsmuscles and underemphasize the muscles that protect your shoulders, such as your posterior deltoids and your trapeziuses.

Of course, this isn't a reason not to lift. The benefits of strength training far outweigh the potential for injury, which can easily be avoided. And aging isn't the culprit, either. A recent survey found that 64 percent of active adults under the age of 45 have joint pains caused by incorrectly lifting weights. That means that if you work out regularly, you're probably in pain or cutting yourself short on gains.

HOT TIP #28

Brew relaxation. In a study at University College in London, 75 men were given tea before completing two stressful tasks. Afterward, their cortisol levels dropped an average of 47 percent, compared with 27 percent for men who weren't given tea.

Now imagine the flip side. What if you made every rep of every set more effective? How much better would you look then? That reality isn't so far-fetched when you consider that your body is no different from a machine. The more efficient you make your movements, the better you'll run. Researchers at the College of New Jersey found that a quick change in bench press technique can instantly boost your bench press by as much as 10 percent. It might not sound like much, but how would you like to go from benching 135 pounds to nearly 150 pounds in one day? That's the power of good form. What's more, Norwegian scientists found that when exercises are done correctly, the incidence of muscle strains is cut by 68 percent and the number of reps you can complete jumps by 17 percent in each set.

But none of this is possible without a formal assessment that points out the areas that need improvement. You can do this with the help of a good trainer, or you can assess and correct your own movements. That's why I designed this simple test, which will have you on track to become *Men's Health* fit faster than ever. As you'll find out in Chapter 3, there are several other measurements that you can use—at any age—to determine just where you stand in terms of your overall health; this assessment focuses instead on your physical capabilities. While there are literally thousands of exercise variations you can perform, a few basic movements serve as the foundation for every exercise.

Mike Robertson, CSCS, a renowned specialist in corrective body work, identified five exercises that will help you assess the areas that you need to improve. Mastering proper form in these exercises will not only help you achieve your goals, but also eliminate the weaknesses and imbalances that lead to your aches and pains. Working the muscles you can't see—like those deep inside your core, hips, and shoulders—can be a difficult process. But target those areas, and your whole body benefits. You'll burn through your workout more efficiently, without pain, and see faster and more dramatic results. And you'll set yourself up for a lifetime of looking, feeling, and living leaner, stronger, and healthier.

The tests in this chapter will establish the baseline level of your fitness. No matter how you perform, don't be discouraged. The exercises in the *Men's Health* Muscle System, Chapter 8, are designed to target all of the movements and muscles in your body and to improve the weaknesses that will be identified in these tests. So whether you have weak abs or poor shoulder stability, the exercises in the *Men's Health* Muscle System will fix problem areas and have you feeling 10 years younger, losing weight, and looking better than ever.

> **HOT TIP #29**
>
> **Shut eye, melt fat.**
> In one study, dieters who slept 8.5 hours a night lost more body fat. Dieters who slept 5.5 hours a night lost more muscle.

After 6 weeks, come back to this initial assessment and retest your ability. Don't be surprised when you pass each test with flying colors and your former self has been replaced with a body worthy of praise. Jason Bourne: You've been warned.

The *Men's Health* Fitness Assessment

Use the five simple exercises on the following pages to learn what areas of your body need strengthening. Read the descriptions, perform the movements, and then have a friend watch you, or look at yourself in the mirror. Use the guide that's with each exercise to assess your performance and determine your weaknesses.

SQUAT TEST

HOW TO DO IT: Stand as tall as you can with your feet spread shoulder-width apart. Lower your body as far as you can by pushing your hips back and bending your knees. Pause, then slowly push yourself back to the starting position.

FRONT VIEW

ASSESS YOUR FORM: As you lower your body to the floor, what are your knees doing? Your hips, knees, and feet should all be in a straight line. If your knees start to cave in toward each other, you're at increased risk for a knee injury. This can be anything from wear and tear that will leave your joints aching to hip weaknesses that predispose you to a serious ligament injury, such as a torn anterior cruciate ligament or meniscus.

YOUR WEAKNESS: Your hips and lateral hamstrings are hip abductors and external rotators. That means they control the movements of your lower limbs, and they keep your knees tracking properly so they don't blow out. You can fix weaknesses in these areas by strengthening your gluteal (butt) and hamstring muscles with exercises like the straight-leg deadlift (see page 176).

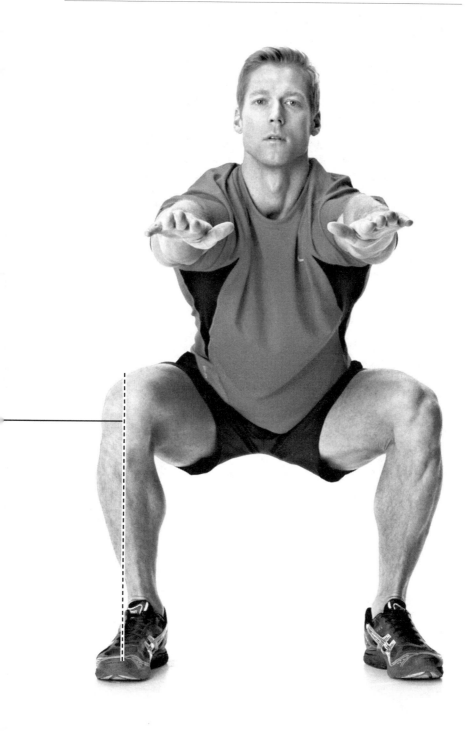

SQUAT TEST

SIDE VIEW

ASSESS YOUR FORM: As you squat, where is your chest positioned? Your chest should remain upright without curving forward.

YOUR WEAKNESS: If you can't keep your chest straight and your shoulders back, it could be indicative of poor thoracic spine extensibility, a weakness in your middle back region. This can lead to neck, shoulder, or lower back pain. You can fix this problem by strengthening your upper back with dumbbell rows (page 185) and the plank and row (page 177), and doing foam-rolling exercises along the upper portion of your back.

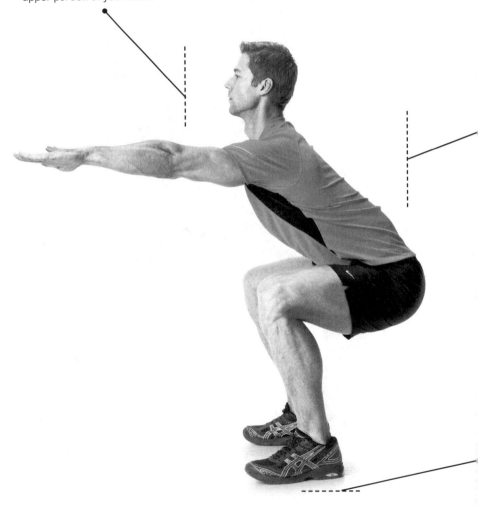

ASSESS YOUR FORM: As you squat, how deep can you go without losing your lower back alignment—that is, keeping your torso upright without rounding your lower back? You should be able to squat until the tops of your thighs are at least parallel to the floor. When you perform the squat with added resistance, the ligaments in your knees are better protected when you lower your thighs below parallel.

YOUR WEAKNESS: If you are unable to get your hips below your knees without rounding your lower back, you need to improve your hip mobility. Over time, poor hip mobility could result in lower back pain. Strengthen your core with an exercise like mountain climbers (page 181), and loosen your hips with foam rolling.

ASSESS YOUR FORM: As you squat, where is your weight balanced? Your body weight should be toward the middle of your foot or on your heels.

YOUR WEAKNESS: If you're on your toes, your quads are too strong in relation to your glutes and hamstrings. A weak backside can lead to low back pain or pain in the fronts of your knees. When you first begin performing the front squat, as shown in the *Men's Health* Muscle System, take a box that comes up to your knees and position it about 2 inches behind your body, then squat so your butt touches the box. This will help you learn to push your hips back. You can strengthen your glutes and hamstrings with dumbbell straight-leg deadlifts (page 176).

LUNGE TEST

HOW TO DO IT: Stand tall with your feet hip-width apart and your hands on your hips. Step forward with your left leg and slowly lower your body until your front knee is bent to at least 90 degrees. Pause, then push yourself to the starting position as quickly as you can. Repeat with your other leg.

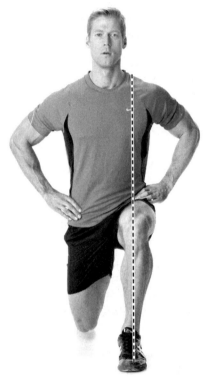

FRONT VIEW

ASSESS YOUR FORM: How do your knee and foot line up as you lower your body? When you're standing, your foot, knee, and hip should be in a straight line. As you lower your body, your knees should remain aligned with the rest of the leg and your thighs should stay oriented with each other.

YOUR WEAKNESS: If your knees cave inward, this could be indicative of weak hip muscles. Weak hips can lead to lower back, hip, or knee pain. Take off your shoes (or wear barefoot shoes like Vibrams) when you perform your lunges. This will help improve stability in your foot, which will ensure better movement in your hips.

SIDE VIEW

ASSESS YOUR FORM: Does your torso move when you perform the lunge? As you complete the movement, your torso should be perpendicular to the floor.

THE WEAKNESS: If your torso leans forward or to the side, you could be too stiff in your hip flexors. Stiff hip flexors often lead to lower back pain or pain in the fronts of your knees. Loosen this area by doing a hip flexor stretch before performing this exercise. Kneel on your left leg, with your right foot on the floor and your right knee bent 90 degrees. Rest your hands on your hips and press your pelvis forward, feeling the stretch in your left hip flexor and quad. Hold for 30 seconds, then repeat on the right side.

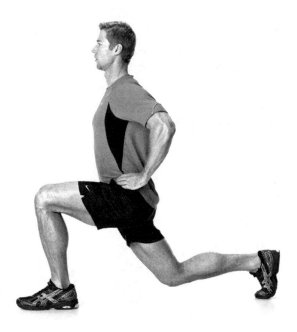

ASSESS YOUR FORM: When you do a lunge, where is your weight balanced? Your body weight should be toward your midfoot or even your heel.

YOUR WEAKNESS: If you're on your toes, your quads are too strong in relation to your glutes and hamstrings. A weak backside could lead to low back pain or pain in the fronts of your knees. When you lunge, make sure you watch yourself in a mirror. Think about standing tall and dropping down straight, rather than rocking forward or backward. If this doesn't work, place a bench a few inches in front of you. This will prevent your knee from drifting forward when you lunge.

PUSHUP TEST

HOW TO DO IT: Get down on all fours and place your hands on the floor so that they're slightly wider than and in line with your shoulders. Straighten your legs, with your weight on your toes. Your body should form a straight line from your head to your ankles. This is your starting position. Lower your body until your chest nearly touches the floor. Pause at the bottom, then push yourself back to the starting position as quickly as possible.

SIDE VIEW

ASSESS YOUR FORM: Does your torso move during the pushup? Your body should be rigid like a board, in a straight line. Your legs should be straight, your stomach and glutes tight, and your chest out.

YOUR WEAKNESS: If your lower back sags as you transition from the lowering to the lifting phase on a pushup, this indicates weak abs or stiff hip flexors. Again, weakness in this region can lead to lower back pain, and can also be improved with incline pushups.

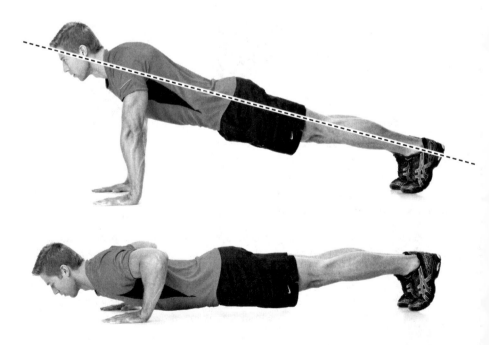

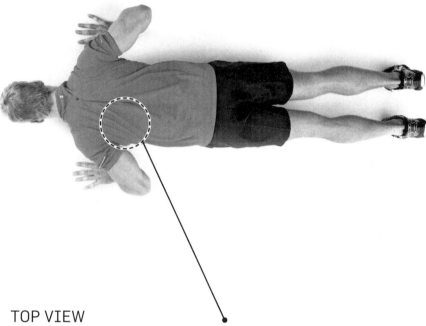

TOP VIEW

ASSESS YOUR FORM: You'll need a friend to watch you on this move. How do your shoulder blades move when you lower your body to the floor? As you perform the pushup, your shoulder blades should move around your rib cage. They shouldn't protrude from your back and be noticeable.

YOUR WEAKNESS: If your shoulder blades are protruding, you have a weak serratus anterior muscle, the "boxer's muscle" that's located on the side of your chest along your ribs; it attaches to and allows you to rotate your shoulder blade. Weakness in your serratus can lead to shoulder pain. Perform incline pushups to improve your pushup form: Place a barbell on the pins of a squat rack at hip height (or set the Smith machine), and perform a pushup. As you improve, gradually lower the bar closer to the floor until you can do the perfect pushup.

FRONT PLANK TEST

HOW TO DO IT: Start to get into a pushup position, but bend your elbows and rest your weight on your forearms instead of on your hands. Your body should form a straight line from your shoulders to your ankles. Brace your core by contracting your abs, as if you are about to be punched in the gut, and hold this position. Count for how many seconds you can hold this optimal alignment. Your eventual goal should be to hold an optimal alignment for 2 minutes.

SIDE VIEW

ASSESS YOUR FORM: Once in position, does any part of your body move? This exercise tests the strength and endurance of your core muscles. Your body should be rigid like a board, forming a straight line from your shoulders to your toes, your stomach and glutes tight, and your chest out.

YOUR WEAKNESS: If you break form in any way, such as raising or sinking your hips, it means your entire core is weak, including your abs, glutes, and even your shoulders. To help perfect your alignment, place a long ruler or a PVC pipe along your back so that it's touching your buttocks, upper back, and the back of your head. The only way to improve your core stabilization is with more planks. Start with a shorter time period, and gradually build your endurance.

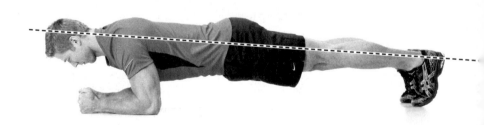

SIDE PLANK TEST

HOW TO DO IT: Lie on your left side with your knees straight. Prop your upper body up on your left elbow and forearm. Brace your core by contracting your abs forcefully, as if you are about to be punched in the gut. Raise your hips until your body forms a straight line from your ankles to your shoulders. Count for how many seconds you can hold this optimal alignment. Your eventual goal should be to hold an optimal alignment for 90 seconds. Switch sides. Be sure to look for differences between the sides.

SIDE VIEW

ASSESS YOUR FORM: How good is your alignment? Your body should be in a straight line and rigid like a board. Your legs should be straight, your belly and glutes tight, and your chest out.

YOUR WEAKNESS: Don't allow your hips to sag toward the floor or drift behind your feet and torso. Failure to keep good alignment indicates weakness in your oblique and trunk muscles. Improve these areas with T-pushups (page 183).

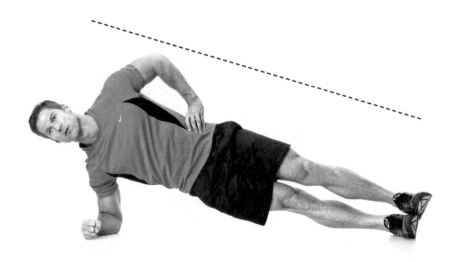

Perfect Your Posture

Even if you follow the *Men's Health* Muscle System to a T, we can't go back in time and eliminate years of poor exercise form or all of the time you spent slumped over your desk, praying for the weekend to arrive. The day-to-day stresses literally change the shape of your body, which can leave you looking more like a hunchback than a hunk. Over time, your poor posture takes a tremendous toll on your spine, shoulders, hips, and knees. In fact, it can cause a cascade of structural flaws that result in acute problems, such as joint pain throughout your body, reduced flexibility, and compromised muscles, all of which can limit your ability to burn fat and build strength.

But don't worry—all of these problems can be corrected. Are you ready to straighten yourself out? Use this head-to-toe guide to make sure your posture is picture-perfect.

Analyze Your Alignment

Strip down to a pair of shorts, and take two full-body photos, one from the front and one from the side. Keep your muscles relaxed, but stand as tall as you can, with your feet hip-width apart. Now compare your photos with those at the right to diagnose your posture problems. Notice the dotted line in the profile phoot. Are your ear, hip, and ankle in alignment? If you spot one of the following problems, add our fixes to your regular workout plan.

DIAGNOSIS

FORWARD HEAD

Your chin protrudes out from your chest and your legs are in front of your shoulders.

WHERE PAIN STRIKES: Neck

THE PROBLEM: Stiff muscles in the back of your neck

FIX IT: Stretch with head nods daily: Moving only your head, drop your chin down and in toward your neck to stretch the back of your neck. Hold for 5 seconds; do this 10 times.

THE PROBLEM: Weak front neck muscles

FIX IT: Do this neck "crunch" every day: Lying faceup on the floor, lift your head so it just clears the floor. Hold for 5 seconds; do 2 or 3 sets of 12 reps daily.

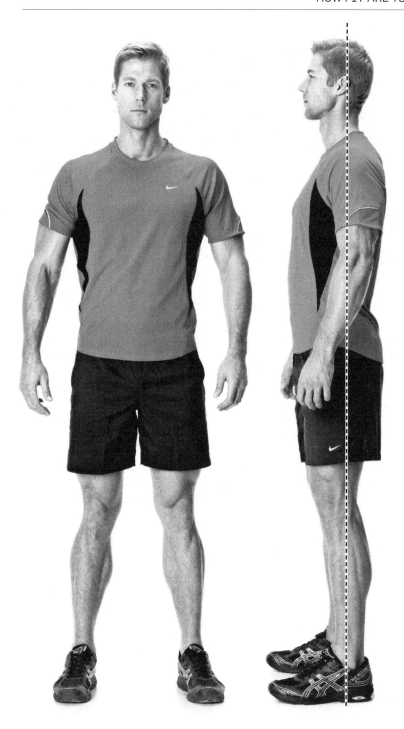

DIAGNOSIS
ELEVATED SHOULDER

Your shoulders are not in line with your collar bone but encroach up toward your ears.

WHERE PAIN STRIKES: Neck and shoulders

THE PROBLEM: A shortened trapezius (the muscle that starts at the back of your neck and runs across your upper back)

FIX IT: Perform an upper-trap stretch. With your higher-side arm behind your back, tilt your head away from your elevated side until you feel the stretch in your upper trapezius. Apply slight pressure with your free hand on your stretched muscle. Hold for 30 seconds; repeat 3 times.

THE PROBLEM: A weak serratus anterior, the muscle just under your pectoral muscles running from your upper ribs to your shoulder blades

FIX IT: Try chair shrugs. Sit upright in a chair with your hands next to your hips, palms down on the seat, and arms straight. Without moving your arms, push down on the chair until your hips lift off the seat and your torso rises. Hold for 5 seconds. That's 1 rep; do 2 or 3 sets of 12 reps daily.

DIAGNOSIS
ROUNDED SHOULDERS

Your shoulders are in front of your hips and ankles instead of in alignment with them.

WHERE PAIN STRIKES: Neck, shoulders, or back

THE PROBLEM: Tight pectoral muscles

FIX IT: Try a simple doorway stretch: Place each forearm against each side of a doorjamb with your elbow bent to 90 degrees. Step through the doorway until you feel the stretch in your chest and the fronts of your shoulders. Hold for 30 seconds. That's 1 set; do 4 daily.

THE PROBLEM: Weakness in the middle and lower parts of your trapezius muscles

FIX IT: Use the floor L raise: Lying facedown on the floor, place each arm at a 90-degree angle in the high-five position—your shoulders, palms, and forearms should all be touching the floor. Without changing your elbow angle, raise both arms by pulling your shoulders back and squeezing your shoulder blades together. Hold for 5 seconds; do 2 or 3 sets of 12 reps daily.

DIAGNOSIS
HUNCHED BACK

Your shoulders are rounded forward and your chest is concave.

WHERE PAIN STRIKES: Neck, shoulders, or back

THE PROBLEM: Poor upper back mobility

FIX IT: Lie faceup on a foam roller placed at about your midback, perpendicular to your spine. Place your hands behind your head and arch your upper back over the roller 5 times. Adjust the roller and repeat on different portions of your upper back.

THE PROBLEM: Weak muscles in your back

FIX IT: Perform the prone cobra. Lie facedown with your arms at your sides, palms down. Lift your head, chest, and hands slightly off the floor, and squeeze your shoulder blades together while keeping your chin tucked. Hold for 5 seconds; do 2 or 3 sets of 12 reps daily.

DIAGNOSIS
ANTERIOR PELVIC TILT

Your lower abdomen protrudes forward and your lower back is arched.

WHERE PAIN STRIKES: Lower back (because of the more pronounced arch in your lumbar spine). The tilt also pushes your belly out, even if you don't have an ounce of belly fat.

THE PROBLEM: Tight hip flexors

FIX IT: Kneel with your right knee on the floor and your left foot flat on the floor in front of you. Tighten your right gluteal muscles until you feel the front of your right hip stretching comfortably. Reach upward with your right arm, and stretch back and to the left. Hold this position for 30 seconds, and repeat 3 times. Switch legs and repeat.

THE PROBLEM: Weak glutes

FIX IT: The glute bridge is your solution. Lie on your back with your knees bent to about 90 degrees. Squeeze your glutes together and push your hips upward until your body is straight from knees to shoulders. Hold for 5 seconds; complete 2 or 3 sets of 12 reps daily.

DIAGNOSIS
PIGEON TOES

One or both feet point slightly inward instead of straight ahead.

WHERE PAIN STRIKES: Knees, hips, or lower back

THE PROBLEM: Tightness in the outer portion of your thigh (your tensor fasciae latae)

FIX IT: Stand up, cross your affected leg behind the other, and lean away from the affected side until you feel your hip stretching comfortably. Hold for 30 seconds. Repeat 3 times.

THE PROBLEM: Weak glutes and medius muscles

FIX IT: Use an exercise called the side-lying clamshell. Lie on one side with your hips and knees bent to 90 degrees and your heels together. Keeping your hips still, raise your top knee upward, separating your knees like a clamshell. Pause for 5 seconds; lower your knee to the starting position. Perform 2 or 3 sets of 12 reps daily.

DIAGNOSIS
DUCK FEET

One or both feet point slightly outward instead of straight ahead.

WHERE PAIN STRIKES: Hips or lower back

THE PROBLEM: You lack flexibility in all the muscles in your hips.

FIX IT: Drop to your hands and knees, and place one foot behind the opposite knee, resting your ankle on the top of your calf. Making sure you keep your spine naturally arched, shift your weight backward and allow your hips to bend until you feel the stretch. Hold the stretch for 30 seconds, repeat 3 times, and then switch sides.

THE PROBLEM: Weakness in your oblique muscles and hip flexors

FIX IT: Try the Swiss-ball jackknife. Assume the top of a pushup position but rest your shins on a Swiss ball. Without rounding your lower back, tuck your knees under your torso by rolling the ball toward your body with your feet. Roll the ball back to the starting position. Do 2 or 3 sets of 12 reps daily.

Mastering proper form will help set you up for a lifetime of looking, feeling, and living leaner, stronger, and healthier.

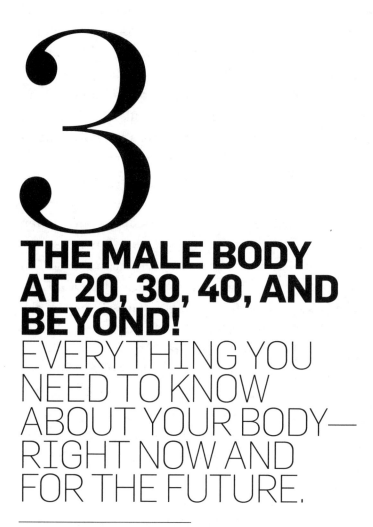

3

THE MALE BODY AT 20, 30, 40, AND BEYOND!

EVERYTHING YOU NEED TO KNOW ABOUT YOUR BODY— RIGHT NOW AND FOR THE FUTURE.

Each and every day of his life, a man makes thousands of decisions. What will I eat for breakfast? What shall I do on my lunch break? The gym after work, or happy hour at 6? Jimmy Kimmel, or a good night's sleep?

Few of these decisions will change the course of a man's life. But day by day, those choices add up to a pattern, one that will reveal itself as the years pass, the way crop circles become apparent the higher up you go in the sky. By the time a man is in his mid-thirties, those decisions may have sculpted him into a classy, perennial champion like Derek Jeter or a washed-up loudmouth like John Rocker (both born in 1974). By the time he's in his late forties, day-to-day choices will determine whether he looks more like square-jawed, hawk-eyed TV pundit Fareed Zakaria or like pie-faced, crocodile-tear-shedding political host Glenn Beck (both circa 1964). A decade or so later, when that same man's turning the corner on 60, he may resemble hard-rocking boss Bruce Springsteen or soft, rocking-chair-bound Billy Joel (each born in 1949). And as he slides into home at about age 80, he may come in tough and lean with a full head of steam like Clint Eastwood (born 1930) or dowdy and doughy with a full face of fat like William Shatner (born a year later, in '31).

> **HOT TIP #30**
>
> **See your way to the gym.** You'll cut your risk of age-related macular degeneration—the leading cause of adult blindness—by 70 percent simply by exercising three times a week, according to a University of Wisconsin study.

You know which of those men you want to be like. You don't want to be that guy who *used to be* a rock star, who *used to be* an athlete, who *used to be* cool and edgy and tough. You want to be that guy who still is, at any age.

Well, you can be.

Winning that battle—the battle to stay at the top of your game—starts with paying attention to health, nutrition, and fitness. It's hard to maintain your edge when all your edges have gone soft and doughy. The *Men's Health* Nutrition System and the *Men's Health* Muscle System are calibrated to strip away fat, starting with your belly first, no matter how old you are or how long that extra weight has been hanging around causing trouble.

But a lot of the battle is also about understanding how your body changes over the first few decades of adulthood and making adjustments in your health and fitness routines so you have the armament you need to carry you into your later years. No matter how fit you are, a health crisis at any point can undermine your best-laid plans. *Men's Health* talked to the world's leading cardiologists, neuroscientists, nutritionists, and trainers to create this guide to your twenties, thirties, forties, and beyond. It can help you anticipate your body's physiological shifts and then guide you through critical adjustments to your lifestyle to match them. Yes, you grow older, but can also grow stronger and even smarter. Here's what you need to know in order to work these changes to your advantage and build the best body you can, no matter what your age.

> **HOT TIP #31**
>
> **Order off the menu.** Most restaurants have healthier choices—brown rice instead of white—that aren't listed on the daily menu. Don't be afraid to ask if there's something better hiding in the kitchen.

Your Twenties

YOUR MUSCLES

In your twenties, you have a wonderful ability to execute intense, heavy, frequent exercise, said Alexander Koch, PhD, an associate professor of exercise science at Truman State University. "Don't blow the opportunity." The reason for that ability: high tides of human growth hormone (HGH) and testosterone—currents that spur the growth of the muscle fibers that ignite explosive lifts, sprints, jumps, and swings. "A man's HGH levels drop from 6 nanograms per milliliter (ng/ml) when he's 20 to 3 ng/ml when he's 40," said Koch. At any age, adding muscle is like putting money in the bank—it will help keep your metabolism high in the coming years, fending off weight gain and diabetes risk. And it will protect you against injury. But as with money, the earlier you can bank it, the greater the long-term payoff.

YOUR PLAN: You should head straight for the heavy weights, said fitness trainer Mike Boyle, ATC. You don't need much cardio because your metabolism still vaporizes pizza on contact. And you don't have to worry about flexibility because your joints are healthy and your range of motion doesn't need priming—yet.

HOT TIP #32

Write it down.
In a 13-week study, dieters who kept a food record for 3 weeks or longer lost 3.5 pounds more than those who didn't, say researchers at the University of Arkansas. To eyeball calories like an expert, log your daily meals for at least 2 weeks on a free Web site like sparkpeople.com.

YOUR SKIN

This is a fairly maintenance-free decade, said David Bank, MD, an author and dermatologist in Mount Kisco, New York. Your skin still has plenty of elastin (the protein that helps skin spring back after stretching) and collagen (the fibrous structural protein that keeps tissue plump).

YOUR PLAN: The bulk of future wrinkles and sun spots are earned before and during this decade, so protect yourself with an oil-free sunscreen with an SPF of 15 or higher. Look for broad-spectrum protection against UVA/UVB rays; products with titanium dioxide and zinc oxide block both. A great way to remember it: Use it every day in place of aftershave balm.

YOUR STRESS LEVEL

The average guy marries at 27. And although I'm sure it's a coincidence, most episodes of major depression start around the same time. Perhaps the cause is a culmination of twentysomething stressors—the kind that come with 70-hour workweeks and late nights on the pub circuit. But it's not just your mind that pays the price. A busy, high-stress lifestyle often leads to a diet of convenience, one that's lacking in vitamins and minerals and overloaded with sugar, fat, and calories. The result: a body that never realizes its full potential.

YOUR PLAN: Eat 1 tablespoon of ground flaxseed daily. It's the best source of alpha-linolenic acid, or ALA—a healthy fat that improves the workings of the cerebral cortex, the area of the brain that processes sensory information, including pleasure, according to nutrition researchers at Hopital Fernand Widal in Paris. Find ground flaxseed in the health food section of your grocery store. To meet your quota, sprinkle it on salads, vegetables, and cereal, or mix it in a smoothie or shake.

HOT TIP #33

Build it with badminton.
Swedish scientists discovered that badminton players saw greater increases in bone density than ice hockey players. Why? In badminton, about 15 percent of your moves are lunges, meaning you're working the large muscles in the legs. Bonus: You get to keep your teeth!

YOUR CANCER RISK

Every hour, your body replicates 6 billion cells by creating copies of your DNA. But if you don't consume enough folate—a B vitamin that helps construct those cells—your body could produce irregular DNA, which can eventually cause cancer, said Ann Yelmokas McDermott, PhD, a nutrition scientist at Tufts University. Trouble is, folate is hard to come by. The best natural food source is chicken liver (yuck), and few men get the folate their bodies require from fruits and vegetables.

YOUR PLAN: The *Men's Health* Nutrition System is designed to boost your intake of vegetables and, hence, folate. But as a backup plan, have a cup of folate-fortified cereal 4 days a week. Choose a brand—such as General Mills's Total Raisin Bran or MultiGrain Cheerios—that provides at least 400 micrograms (mcg) of folate per serving. Then top it with a cup of blackberries, raspberries, or strawberries. Berries aren't just a good nonliver source of folate; they're packed with antioxidants, which help thwart cancer by neutralizing DNA-damaging free radicals.

YOUR BONES

Bones are a lot like reclusive co-workers: Until one snaps, you aren't likely to give them much thought. But this is your last chance to lay down new bone; by the time you're 30, your skeletal system is set. Poor nutrition not only inhibits your ability to grow bone, but also increases your risk of disease, weight gain, and cognitive decline—now and for decades down the road.

HOT TIP #34

Mate (again and again) for life.
A study of 1,000 middle-age subjects found that those who had frequent orgasms had a 50 percent lower death rate. Can we get a prescription for that?

YOUR PLAN: Drink two 8-ounce glasses of vitamin D–fortified milk every day. This provides your body with 600 milligrams (mg) of calcium and 5 mcg of vitamin D, the perfect combination of nutrients to build break-resistant bones. Plus, in a 20-year study, U.K. researchers determined that men who drink more than 6 ounces of milk a day have half the risk of stroke as men who drink less.

YOUR JEWELS

Testicular cancer is the most common form of the disease in men ages 15 to 34. It also has one of the highest 5-year survival rates—more than 90 percent, according to the American Cancer Society. Of course, you have to catch it first, and since pain is only occasionally a symptom, it's critical that you perform self-examinations regularly.

YOUR PLAN: Once a month, look for abnormal swelling and use your thumbs and index fingers to feel for lumps, which are usually the size of a pea. It helps if you perform the test after a warm shower, when your scrotum is relaxed.

YOUR HIV STATUS

Twenty percent of the estimated 1 million Americans infected with HIV don't know they're infected, so they aren't taking medicines to suppress it, according to the Centers for Disease Control and Prevention (CDC). That's why they recommend that everyone—even those in low-risk groups—be screened for the disease at an annual exam.

YOUR PLAN: The best tests are the HIV ELISA and Western blot, which you should get once every 5 years starting in your twenties. The HIV ELISA (enzyme-linked immunosorbent assay) requires a blood sample, but oral swabs are an option for the needle-phobic. A second test, the Western blot, is needed to confirm those results because other conditions, such as lupus, Lyme disease, and syphilis, can produce a false positive ELISA result. The FDA has also approved a do-it-yourself kit called Home Access HIV-1, which allows you to send a prick of blood to a private lab for confidential testing.

YOUR BLOOD SUGAR LEVEL

The American Diabetes Association estimates that one-third of all men with type 2 diabetes don't know they're diabetic. What's more, most of them could have avoided the condition altogether with pre-

> **HOT TIP #35**
>
> **Listen to smoothie jazz.** Whey protein not only helps you build muscle, but it boosts your body's production of glutathione, an antioxidant that University of Buffalo researchers found could limit noise-induced hearing loss in mice.

ventive screening. "If your fasting blood glucose is in a prediabetic range [between 100 and 125 mg/per deciliter (dl)], you can prevent the disease with lifestyle changes," said David Johnson, PhD, coauthor of *Medical Tests That Can Save Your Life.*

YOUR PLAN: A study in the *New England Journal of Medicine* found that exercising for 30 minutes a day and losing 5 percent of your body weight by eating a diet rich in fruits, vegetables, and fiber could reduce your risk of developing diabetes by 58 percent. You should get a fasting blood glucose test once a year starting in your twenties.

YOUR TEETH

There's a strong link between periodontal disease and blood markers for heart disease. "When oral bacteria travel through the bloodstream, they can cause the liver to pump out CRP [C-reactive protein, a marker for inflammation]," said Brent Bauer, MD, professor of medicine at the Mayo Clinic. "The inflammation that results may be a factor in causing atherosclerosis." Fortunately, gum disease is usually reversible if caught early.

YOUR PLAN: Get a dental exam and cleaning twice a year starting in your twenties.

YOUR BELLY

Nearly three-quarters of American men are overweight or obese, but only 5 percent recognize that they have a problem, according to a recent Pew Research Survey. Ignorance can be deadly. Studies

---

HOT TIP #36

Prolong your workout. When you're in the middle of a run or bike ride, and you feel like hanging it up, take a deep breath and blow out hard. This mind-clearing technique is known as the "explosive exhale." It allows you to "blow out all your demons," says Amby Burfoot, former Boston Marathon champion and contributing editor of *Runner's World.*

associate weight gain with a host of diseases, including high blood pressure, diabetes, heart disease, and even cancer.

YOUR PLAN: Use the body mass index (BMI), which estimates body fat based on your height and weight, to determine if you're in the danger zone (visit menshealth.com/ mhdiet for a quick-and-easy BMI calculator). Measure yourself every 3 years, or whenever you gain weight, starting in your twenties. A score between 18.5 and 24.9 is normal. BMI doesn't take into account muscle mass, though, so if you're lifting weights often (as you should), use the U.S. Navy circumference method for measuring body fat (you'll find it, too, at menshealth.com/mhdiet). You'll need to take a few measurements, but you'll get a more accurate reading.

> **HOT TIP #37**
>
> **Pop one for productivity.**
> Taking a multivitamin could make you a better multitasker, say UK researchers. Try a multi with a 300 percent daily value (DV) of vitamin B6, 150 percent DV of folic acid, and 50 percent DV of vitamin B12.

YOUR LIFE

According to the CDC, "unintentional injuries" is the number one cause of death for men in their twenties.

YOUR PLAN: Be careful out there, people. To paraphrase Jeff Foxworthy, you don't want your last words to be "Hey, watch this . . . !"

Your Thirties

YOUR MUSCLES

You may find that you can't lift as much weight as you could in your twenties, because your testosterone level begins to drop about 1 percent a year once you hit the big 3-0. That means it will take longer for your muscles to return to full strength after each workout.

YOUR PLAN: Eat broccoli and bell peppers. Together, they're packed with vitamins C and E, two nutrients that fight free radicals—rogue molecules that slow the repair of exercise-induced muscle damage, impeding recovery.

YOUR SKIN

This is a transitional decade for your skin. You've kind of passed your peak oil moment, facewise: Oil production drops about 10 percent in this decade, and the skin thins about the same amount. Prior sun damage crops up in the forms of crow's-feet; and skin sags, thanks to collagen loss. A late night is far more likely to bring out dark circles, bags, and puffiness.

YOUR PLAN: If you like to work out alfresco, try to schedule exercise for before 10 a.m. or after 4 p.m. Sweating exposes your skin to salt water, which can break down the skin's defenses and allow more ultraviolet light and pollutants to reach skin cells. Staying out of the sunlight in the late morning and early afternoon can eliminate 80 percent of UVB penetration. And remember, you don't have to be a hipster to wear a straw hat on sunny summer days. It will protect your face as well as any thinning real estate up top.

HOT TIP #38

Mix and max.
To maximize gains, vary reps and the amount of weight you lift. Muscles grow when they are forced to adapt. A recent study in the *Journal of Strength and Conditioning Research* found that men who regularly varied their reps increased their bench strength by 28 percent and their leg-press strength by 43 percent.

YOUR METABOLISM

The metabolic rate that allowed you to burn through supersize burritos in your twenties is slowing—dropping by 1 percent every 4 years. The likely reason: Lower testosterone is making it harder for you to build—or even maintain—metabolism-boosting muscle.

YOUR PLAN: Keep lifting. "As you strengthen your muscles, the amount of testosterone your body produces increases," said David Zava, PhD, CEO of ZRT Laboratory. But be realistic about both the weight you're lifting and how often you do it. You need to push iron only twice a week to see the benefit. So, make sure active rest is part of your fitness strategy. (For some great ideas on boosting fitness outside the gym, see page 201.)

YOUR JOINTS

Even though arthritis doesn't usually set in until your fifties, the damage that causes it, cartilage degeneration, happens in your thirties.

YOUR PLAN: Eat 6-ounces of coldwater fish three times a week. Specifically, have salmon, mackerel, trout, or white tuna—each packs more than 1,000 mg of fish oil. A U.K. study found that regularly consuming this amount of fish oil appeared to halt cartilage-eating enzymes in 86 percent of people who were facing joint replacement surgery. Fish oil slows down cartilage degeneration and reduces factors that cause inflammation, said lead researcher Bruce Caterson, PhD.

YOUR BLOOD PRESSURE

Starting at age 30, your systolic blood pressure rises 4 points per decade. (Probably more if you spend too much time watching Fox News or MSNBC.) Researchers from the Netherlands recently discovered that besides the obvious factors—obesity, lack of physical activity, and high salt consumption—diets containing too little potassium were the primary cause of hypertension. In their analysis, the scientists used 3,500 mg daily as the cutoff for defining a "low" potassium

> **HOT TIP #39**
>
> **Pencil it in.**
> Schedule your workout like you schedule any meeting. If your assistant makes appointments for your business lunches, ask him or her to schedule your workouts as well.

intake. That's bad news because the average American man in his thirties gets only 3,100 mg a day.

YOUR PLAN: Add ½ cup of beans, a banana, or a handful of raisins to your daily diet. Each will increase your potassium intake by about 400 mg a day, boosting you above that 3,500 mg benchmark.

And don't forget to test your blood pressure once a year. A reading below 120/80 mm Hg is desirable, and anything over 140/90 mm Hg is cause for concern. If yours falls between these numbers, take note: You have prehypertension, which means you're likely to develop high blood pressure if you don't start taking preventive action now.

YOUR HEART

Fifty percent of heart attacks occur in people with normal levels of LDL cholesterol (the bad kind). So if you're in a high-risk group because of race, blood pressure, or family history, you might benefit from asking your doctor for some additional blood tests.

> **HOT TIP #40**
>
> **Tag-team your weight loss.**
> Work out with a friend and you'll exercise for an additional 34 minutes, according to the American College of Sports Medicine. And researchers at the University of Oxford found that men who trained in a group tolerated pain better than those who exercised alone.

YOUR PLAN: The high-sensitivity CRP test looks for elevated levels of C-reactive protein, which is produced by your liver in response to inflammation and is as predictive of heart disease as high cholesterol. Homocysteine is an amino acid, and elevated levels often signal the buildup of plaque, cholesterol, and calcium in your arteries, said Stanley Hazen, MD, PhD, director of the Cleveland Clinic's Center for Cardiovascular Diagnostics and Prevention. And at least once every 5 years, starting in your twenties, you should have a full lipid profile test. Unlike common cholesterol screens, this blood

THE TESTS OF TIME

Five fast ways to determine if you're aging gracefully

HEARING

THE TEST: Go to freemosquitoringtones.org and see if you can hear the ring tone appropriate for your age.

SIGNS OF A PROBLEM: If certain consonant sounds, such as C, D, K, P, S, and T, are hard to distinguish, see a hearing specialist.

WHAT TO DO: Include lean meat, dairy and leafy greens in your diet. Lack of vitamin B_{12} and folate have been linked to age-related hearing loss.

EYESIGHT

THE TEST: How far away is your book? It should be less than an arm's length away.

SIGNS OF A PROBLEM: Having to hold reading material farther away than you used to in order to see it is a sign of age-related vision loss.

WHAT TO DO: When reading, make sure you are comfortable with the lighting. Eat carrots and kale, which are high in vision-boosting vitamin A and lutein.

MEMORY

THE TEST: You should be able to remember up to seven random numbers after seeing them for only 3 seconds.

SIGNS OF A PROBLEM: Forgetting where you put your keys is normal. Not knowing what your keys are used for isn't.

WHAT TO DO: Challenge your brain with puzzles, stay physically active, and go out often with your friends to keep you mentally sharp.

BALANCE

THE TEST: You should be able to close your eyes, stand on one leg, and hold your raised leg to your chest for 30 seconds without hopping around.

SIGNS OF A PROBLEM: If you trip, slip, and bump into things on a daily basis or often feel dizzy or light-headed, you should see a doctor.

WHAT TO DO: Tai chi improves muscle coordination and blood circulation while increasing muscle strength and tone.

MUSCLE MASS

THE TEST: You should be able to do 8 squats and 2 sets of 8 pushups.

SIGNS OF A PROBLEM: Sarcopenia, the age-related loss of muscle mass, progresses slowly and almost imperceptibly.

WHAT TO DO: Follow the *Men's Health* Muscle System—in Chapter 8.

test measures the levels of four different kinds of blood fats: LDL cholesterol, HDL cholesterol, very-low-density lipoprotein (VLDL), and triglycerides. It provides a clearer picture of circulatory health and helps your physician pinpoint any problems, said Thomas Owens, MD, chief medical officer of Duke University Hospital.

YOUR SEX DRIVE

A dropping testosterone level, coupled with a rising stress level, can put a crimp in a man's mojo. You need to protect the beast.

YOUR PLAN: Munch on two handfuls of walnuts, peanuts, or almonds every day. Research shows that men with diets high in monounsaturated fat—the kind found in nuts—have higher testosterone levels than those who don't eat enough of the healthy fat. Nuts are also the best food source of arginine, an amino acid that improves bloodflow throughout your body—including below the belt.

HOT TIP #41

Make 1+1=3. Order broccoli on pizza, or puree and add it to pasta sauce. In studies, the combo of broccoli and tomatoes has been shown to shrink prostate cancer cells faster and more effectively than any other treatment except castration. (Bet that enhances the appeal, huh?)

YOUR BELLY

From his thirties on, the average guy starts to add on adipose tissue (a.k.a. flab). Your metabolism slows and your body-fat percentage creeps up. More than any other measure, your body-fat percentage indicates your overall health.

YOUR PLAN: Work to keep your BMI below 22 (18 is optimal). Research shows that doing this reduces your risk of high blood pressure, diabetes, and heart disease. Eating the right breakfast—one with lots of protein—will keep your belly at bay, according to multiple studies on the subject. (This is such an important aspect of weight management that the *Men's Health* Rules of the Ripped include an emphasis on always, always eating breakfast.) The protein is key: People on weight-loss diets who break eggs for breakfast, for instance, lose 65 percent more weight than those who down a bagel with the same number of calories, according to a study in the *International Journal of Obesity*.

YOUR BACK

As you grow older, you should begin to decrease spinal loading when you work out.

YOUR PLAN: Protect your back by replacing high-weight, low-rep lifts with lower-weight, higher-rep sets and doing some exercises on one leg to iron out muscle imbalances. Doing more reps with a lighter load still yields benefits, but with less structural stress. Include Swiss-ball rollouts, which help you build core strength and endurance. (Sit on your knees and place forearms and fists on the ball. Slowly roll the ball forward, straightening your arms without allowing your lower back to collapse. Then use your abs to pull the ball back to your knees.) In fact, men with poor muscular endurance in their lower backs are three times as likely to develop back pain as those with fair or good endurance, according to a study in *Clinical Biomechanics*.

> **HOT TIP #42**
>
> **Don't drain in vain.** The clear liquid on the top of yogurt is pure whey protein—the stuff they charge you $5 a pop for at the gym. Don't drain it off, just stir it back in and enjoy.

YOUR STRESS LEVEL

After a man turns 30, a new set of stressors tends to emerge: family, a mortgage, and rising job responsibilities, to name a few. And sure enough, levels of the stress hormone cortisol go up. Cortisol is the belly-fat hormone: It can actually blunt the body's production of testosterone and cause your gut to grow.

YOUR PLAN: Log on to funnyordie.com. It doesn't matter if the first video you find is any good or not: Even the anticipation of a good laugh decreases the stress chemicals cortisol and epinephrine by 39 and 70 percent, respectively, said researchers at Loma Linda University. Laughter is also great for the heart. When participants in a University of Maryland study watched stressful film clips, they experienced vasoconstriction, a narrowing of the blood vessels. But the blood vessels of those watching funny films expanded by 22 percent. That's great news—unless you're a Scorsese fan.

HOT TIP #43

Drop weight by raisin it. The raisins in commercial raisin brans are typically coated with sugar. Buy wheat flakes and add your own dried fruits. You'll save 7 grams of sugar—enough to lose 5 pounds in a year if you do it every day.

YOUR LIFE

Oncoming traffic is the number one killer of men in their thirties. "Men in this age group are drinking and driving less, but they're traveling more frequently for work," said Alexander Weiss, PhD, previously director of the Northwestern University Center for Public Safety. "And they still enjoy driving fast and have a tendency to drive aggressively."

YOUR PLAN: Turn off your cell phone when you're behind the wheel. Up to 50 percent of fatal traffic accidents are caused by driver distraction, according to AAA, and just the ping! of an arriving text message can cause you to take your eyes off the road. And beware the danger hour: Researchers at Carnegie Mellon University determined that fatal accidents are most likely to occur between 2 a.m. and 3 a.m. "During the early morning hours, your body is programmed to sleep," said Anne T. McCartt, PhD, senior vice president of research at the Insurance Institute for Highway Safety. So don't be afraid to pull over and nap. Better a little nap now than the big sleep before your time.

5 EASY WAYS
TO INCREASE YOUR MANPOWER

As if losing muscle mass, bone density, and your sex drive to a low testosterone level wasn't bad enough, new research shows that a decline in the male hormone can also increase your risk of prostate cancer and heart disease. Follow these steps to both strengthen and lengthen your life.

1 UNCOVER YOUR ABS
As your waist size goes up, your testosterone goes down. In fact, a 4-point increase in your body mass index—about 30 extra pounds on a 5-foot-10 guy—can accelerate your age-related T decline by 10 years.

2 BUILD YOUR BICEPS
Finnish researchers recently found that men who lifted weights regularly experienced a 49 percent boost in their free testosterone levels. You need to push iron at least twice a week to see the benefit.

3 DON'T FORGET THE FAT
Trimming lard from your diet can help you stay lean, but eliminating all fat can cause your T levels to plummet. A study published in the *International Journal of Sports Medicine* revealed that men who consumed the most fat also had the highest T levels. To protect your heart and preserve your T, add in more foods high in monounsaturated fats, such as fish and nuts. Most men don't get enough of them.

4 PUSH AWAY FROM THE BAR
Happy hour can wreak havoc on your manly hormones. In a recent Dutch study, men who drank moderate amounts of alcohol daily for 3 weeks experienced a 7 percent decrease in their testosterone levels. Limit your drinking to one or two glasses of beer or wine a night to avoid a drop in T.

5 STRIP AWAY STRESS
Mental or physical stress can quickly depress your T levels. Stress causes cortisol to surge, which "suppresses the body's ability to make testosterone and utilize it within tissues," said Dr. Zava. Cardio can be a great tension tamer, unless you overdo it. Injuries and fatigue are signs that your workout is more likely to lower T than raise it.

Your Forties and Beyond

YOUR SEX LIFE

There's no better way to feel like a 20-year-old than to have sex like one (or with one, really). But plaque buildup affects bloodflow in the small arteries of a man's penis sooner than anywhere else in his body, according to Steven Lamm, MD, an internist and the author of *The Hardness Factor*. That's one reason the angle of a man's erection falls to 100 degrees by age 45, down from 130 degrees in his twenties.

YOUR PLAN: Eat as many servings of fruits and vegetables as you can every day. Consider one serving to be ½ cup of cooked spinach, broccoli, or brussels sprouts. They help lower your cholesterol level, an improvement that combats cardiovascular disease and increases bloodflow to the penis. Leafy green vegetables are excellent sources of folate, calcium, magnesium, and zinc. Citrus fruits offer plenty of vitamin C. Go heavy on the blueberries. They're the fruit with the highest amounts of free-radical-crushing antioxidants. And put a little kick in your food with chili peppers, ginger, and other spices, which can enhance sexual performance by increasing circulation.

> **HOT TIP #44**
>
> **Go into the light.** Exercising in direct sunlight helps you lose up to 20 percent more body fat by boosting the appetite-killing hormone leptin.

YOUR MUSCLES

The average guy loses 6 pounds of muscle by the time he's 49. And a lot of that muscle loss comes simply from neglect—skipping the gym literally causes you to replace muscle with fat, according to a study published in the *Journal of the American College of Nutrition*.

That's particularly problematic, because a pound of fat takes up 18 percent more space on your body than a pound of muscle does. So even if you weigh the same as you did on your wedding day, you may not be as appealingly shaped as you once were.

YOUR PLAN: In addition to lifting weights, you can protect your hard-earned muscles by feeding them the right foods. Ounce for ounce, tuna is one of the best sources of muscle-boosting protein—and it contains zero saturated fat. Spinach can help with muscle maintenance. Recent test-tube research from Rutgers, The State University of New Jersey found that a hormone in spinach increases protein synthesis. Spinach is also rich in vitamin K, potassium, and calcium, which can help you ward off osteoporosis.

YOUR JOINTS

Your nerve fibers are losing their effectiveness, which diminishes coordination. Your heart beats more slowly, cutting down the bloodflow that delivers nutrients to and removes waste from joints and muscles. And that's on top of the fact that you're losing about 0.5 percent of your muscle mass a year. As a result, your joints are becoming more vulnerable to injury and to the onset of arthritis.

YOUR PLAN: Your workouts should emphasize flexibility. "Yoga is especially beneficial for men in their forties, because that's when flexibility declines more," says Mehmet Oz, MD, a professor of surgery at Columbia University and coauthor of *You: The Owner's Manual.* New science shows that doing yoga can improve flexibility, relieve back pain, and reduce stress. Boston University researchers reported that

> **HOT TIP #45**
>
> **Be wind blown.**
> When you're cycling or running, start out with the wind behind you and return facing the wind. This way you get a boost when you're cold. Wind in your face is more tolerable once you've warmed up.

people who did yoga weekly boosted levels of the antianxiety brain chemical GABA, or gamma-aminobutyric acid, by 27 percent. Practicing yoga can also help your body maintain its antioxidant levels, which become depleted when you're run down, reported Indian researchers.

YOUR SKIN

In your forties, crow's-feet become creases, and expression lines on your forehead are more difficult to ignore. The loss of tissue under the eyes may produce a hollow look. Moisture production drops another 10 percent, and collagen continues to plummet, causing additional wrinkles to form.

YOUR PLAN: Soothe parched skin with extra emollients overnight. Look for a night cream that lists one of these active ingredients: retinol (vitamin A), antioxidants, vitamin C, or peptides.

YOUR SKIN CANCER RISK

Scientists at the University of California at Irvine discovered that men over 40 were up to twice as likely to develop melanomas than were women of the same age.

YOUR PLAN: Examine your skin for the ABCDs of birthmarks and moles: Asymmetrical, Borders with ragged edges, Color changes, or Diameters bigger than 6 millimeters. If you've spent a lot of time in the sun or gone 5 years without a professional exam, ask your doctor to look you over. And protect yourself by eating smarter. National Cancer Institute researchers determined that people with the highest intakes of carotenoids—pigments that occur naturally in plants—were as much as six times less likely to develop

> **HOT TIP #46**
>
> **Count backward.**
> When you're counting repetitions, start with your target number and count backward—you'll be thinking how few you have left instead of how many you've done.

skin cancer than those with the lowest intakes. Eat two servings of sweet potatoes, carrots, or cantaloupe every week. This will pack your diet with the same amount of weekly beta-carotene as those of men who demonstrated the lowest skin cancer risk had.

YOUR VISION

You were first warned about going blind as a teen; this time, the threat is real.

YOUR PLAN: The National Institutes of Health found that people who consume the most lutein—a carotenoid found in plant foods—are 43 percent less likely to develop macular degeneration. Lutein helps filter blue light, preventing it from damaging retinal tissues. Eat two servings of greens each day. Once every 2 years, get a glaucoma (tonometry) test; by 2020, the number of people over age 40 with diag-noed cases of glaucoma will reach 3.3 million, according to the National Eye Institute. A simple eye exam—which looks for symptoms such as increased eye pressure and general vision deterioration—is all it takes to catch the disease early.

> **HOT TIP #47**
>
> **Take tea for teeth.** Researchers in Japan assessed the drinking habits of some 25,000 adults and found that those who drank at least a cup of green tea a day had a lower risk of tooth loss than those who drank none.

YOUR PROSTATE

Thirty percent of men in their forties have asymptomatic prostate cancer, according to research from the Barbara Ann Karmanos Cancer Institute. That is, the cancer is there but nearly undetectable. Do not freak out: That doesn't mean that you'll develop full-blown cancer, only that you need to be wise about protecting yourself.

YOUR PLAN: Harvard researchers found that men with the highest intake of selenium had a 48 percent lower incidence of advanced prostate cancer than those with the lowest intakes. Simple fix: Eat three Brazil nuts every day. That'll provide you with 200 mcg of selenium, the exact amount you need to keep your prostate cancer risk at rock-bottom levels. Mushrooms help, too: A half cup of the cooked fungi—specifically, brown and portobello—contains more than 35 mcg, or nearly 20 percent of the amount you need daily. Researchers at the Fred Hutchinson Cancer Research Center in Seattle found that men who ate three or more servings of cruciferous vegetables (arugula, broccoli, cauliflower) a week had a 41 percent lower risk of prostate cancer than those who ate just one. Plus, once a year you should have a PSA test. This blood test measures your level of prostate-specific antigen (PSA); an increase of more than 0.75 over 1 year indicates a higher risk of prostate cancer and should be further evaluated. To ensure accurate results: (1) Make sure your doctor takes into account the size of your prostate, as the gland grows larger and produces more PSA over time, and (2) ask how much of the antigen is "free floating." Men with prostate cancer have less of the free variety.

> **HOT TIP #48**
>
> **Sleep or workout?**
> Sleep! "If you're sleep deprived and not just groggy, stay in bed," says Alan Aragon, MS, a nutritionist in Thousand Oaks, California. University of Chicago researchers found that lack of sleep packs on pounds by slowing metabolism and increasing your appetite.

YOUR HEART

Until age 44, accidents are the most likely cause of death in men. But once you reach 45, heart disease becomes your number one threat, killing 36,000 fortysomething men every year. "These men don't consider themselves vulnerable, so they ignore the warning signs," said Richard Stein, MD, professor of cardiology at New York University Langone Medical Center in New York City.

YOUR PLAN: With proper conditioning (high-intensity activities such as circuit training work best), you can increase your heart's stroke volume and your body's oxygen uptake. This allows your heart to pump blood more slowly and efficiently. "The average human life span is about 3 billion heartbeats," said Michael Lauer, MD, of the National Heart, Lung, and Blood Institute. "If you can lower your resting heart rate, you can increase your life expectancy." It's that simple. (The *Men's Health* Muscle System will raise your heart rate into the aerobic zone even as it's helping you build and protect muscle, making your heart more efficient and improving your cardiovascular health.) To check in on the health of your heart, get a 64-slice CT scan once you reach 40, then every 5 years or as necessary, depending on results. The 64-slice CT scan records images so fast that it captures your heart between beats and renders it in 3-D, providing a clearer picture of your coronary arteries than any other type of scan. It detects hard and soft plaques in arteries and gauges your risk of having a heart attack in the future.

> **HOT TIP #49**
>
> **Gobble more.** Substituting turkey for beef or pork slashes an average of 108 calories per meal.

YOUR STROKE RISK

Strokes are the third-leading cause of death in the United States. Eighty percent of all strokes are due to blood clots caused by plaque, and half the time, your first symptom is your last.

YOUR PLAN: Get a carotid duplex ultrasound once at age 40, then as necessary, depending on results. This noninvasive 10-minute test could show if you're at risk. It provides two views of the arteries in your neck, which reveal damage from plaque buildup and how that damage is affecting bloodflow to your brain. This test isn't normally covered by insurance, but you can get it for less than $100 at a handful of private companies.

YOUR COLON

Colon cancer is the third-most-common type of cancer among men and the second-leading cause of cancer-related death, but recent studies indicate that most men have never been screened for it. There's good reason to catch it early: The survival rate is 93 percent if the cancer is treated before it spreads beyond the colon's walls.

YOUR PLAN: Of all the tests used to screen for colon cancer, the colonoscopy is the gold standard. The problem with most other tests is that either they don't examine the colon directly (the fecal occult blood test, for example, analyzes your stool for blood) or they don't reach far enough inside your colon. It's a big organ, and half of all colon cancers occur in the half that's not examined by a sigmoidoscope. A colonoscopy, however, examines every inch, right up to the small intestine. If you have a history of colorectal cancer in your family, schedule this test about 10 years earlier than the age of your relative when he or she was first diagnosed, or in your early forties if there's no family history.

As your waist size goes up, your testosterone goes down, but men who lift weights get a 49 percent boost in T levels.

ANATOMY OF A POTBELLY (AND FIVE REASONS YOU MIGHT STILL BE FAT.)

There are two kinds of potbellies—soft ones and hard ones. And which kind you have may make all the difference in how long, and how well, you're going to live.

The best way to understand the difference is to imagine that a sumo wrestler is bearing down on you. The deafening rumble of the

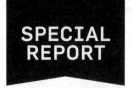
mat below his feet is caused by the weight of all that fat, which is jiggling up and down as he rushes closer, ready to snap your spine like a matchstick. How can he be so strong, and so fast, if he's so fat?

Because of the kind of fat he's carrying.

According to a Japanese study published in the *International Journal of Sports Medicine*, the fat on the bellies of sumo wrestlers is almost entirely *subcutaneous*. That means it's located just under the skin, in front of the abdominal muscles—which is why the wrestlers' bellies jiggle around like Jell-O during an earthquake. Most American men, however, have a very different kind of potbelly—solid and round, as if we swallowed a hard hat or a miniature Volkswagen Beetle. (Think of Hank from *King of the Hill*: He has the kind of body a lot of men have, soft in the shoulders but solid around the belt line.) A belly like that is composed of visceral fat, which resides behind the abdominal muscles, surrounding your internal organs (the viscera). That fat pushes the abdominal muscles outward, making them protrude into a hard, round gut.

And over the past decade, scientists have concluded that the rounder and harder your belly, the more it puts your health in danger.

For that to make sense, it's important to understand that fat—any fat, subcutaneous or visceral—isn't just lifeless tissue whose only duty is to make you cringe at the idea of taking your shirt off in public. "Fat is an endocrine organ that secretes numerous substances, collectively called 'adipokines,' many of which are harmful," says Robert

> **HOT TIP #50**
>
> **Bookmark this.** Users of an online weight-loss program dropped between 11 and 16 pounds when they were sent e-mail encouragements, compared with just a 6-pound drop among the unprodded, says a study in the *Archives of Internal Medicine*. Sign up for weekly reminders at menshealth.com.

Ross, PhD, an exercise physiologist at Queen's University in Canada who's been studying the effects of lifestyle on visceral fat for 18 years. Adipokines include resistin, a hormone that leads to high blood sugar; angiotensinogen, a compound that raises blood pressure; adiponectin, a hormone that regulates the metabolism of lipids and glucose (amounts of this hormone decrease with increased visceral fat); and interleukin-6, a chemical associated with arterial inflammation. And because visceral fat is significantly more active than subcutaneous fat, it produces more of these hazardous secretions. Size also matters: The larger a visceral fat cell grows, the more active it becomes.

You might liken the difference between subcutaneous and visceral fat to that between a dormant volcano and one that's active. The latter is spewing out nasty stuff all the time; the former is just part of the landscape.

YOUR METABOLISM UNDER ATTACK

Now, here's what all this means to you: If your belly is bulging with visceral fat, it's likely that you have the beginnings of something called metabolic syndrome. Metabolic syndrome is a condition that's diagnosed when a man is afflicted with a cluster of heart-disease risk factors—specifically, a 40-inch (or greater) waist, high triglycerides (the fat in your blood), high blood sugar, low HDL cholesterol (the good kind), and high blood pressure, according to the American Heart Association. This combination increases the likelihood you'll develop diabetes by 500 percent, have a heart attack by 300 percent, and die of a heart attack by 200 percent. (Become diabetic, and there's an 80 percent chance you'll die of heart disease.)

And that brings us back to the sumo who's now launching his 400-pound self at you.

Despite having waists that far exceed 40 inches, most sumos

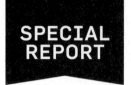
don't exhibit any of the three blood markers for metabolic syndrome—high triglycerides, high blood sugar, or low HDL cholesterol. Again, it comes down to the jiggle factor—more subcutaneous fat, less visceral fat, less risk of diabetes and heart disease. So that prompts the question: How do you know whether your belly houses dangerous levels of visceral fat or if you have the internal makeup of a sumo wrestler?

The first step is to take that waist measurement. If it's approaching 40 inches, your immediate plan of action—besides a new diet and exercise regimen—should be a visit to the doctor. There, you'll want to request a full "metabolic profile." If you have an increasing waistline and any two of the aforementioned requirements for metabolic syndrome, you most assuredly have high amounts of visceral fat. It's more likely than you think probably: Recent estimates suggest that metabolic syndrome affects nearly 17 percent of men over 20, and more than 40 percent of men over 40.

Unlike subcutaneous fat, visceral fat can't be liposuctioned away. But it's also easier to target by less invasive means. Some easy strategies:

> **HOT TIP #51**
>
> **Outrun hunger.**
> Tame cravings with exercise. A British study found that after 58 people worked out every day for 12 weeks, they rated identical breakfasts as 24 percent more filling than they had at the start of the trial. Excercise may raise levels of hormones that affect fullness, says study author Neil King, PhD.

BUT HAVE JUST ONE DRINK FIRST In a study at the University at Buffalo, the men with the most visceral fat drank only once or twice every 2 weeks but consumed more than four drinks each time. Those with the least visceral fat, on the other hand, drank small amounts of alcohol every day—usually about one drink.

TARGET VISCERAL FAT WITH THIS BELLY-BUSTING WORKOUT

Here's how to flatten your gut in less than 30 minutes, 3 times a week

1 WEIGHT WORKOUT

We've given you four upper body exercises, two lower body exercises, and two core (abs and lower back) exercises. Do them as a circuit—performing one after the other with no rest in between—but arrange them so that you alternate upper body exercises with those for your lower body and core. Resting and working your muscles in this way will allow you to work harder in less time, said Jean-Paul Francoeur, owner of JP Fitness, a health club in Little Rock, Arkansas.

Try this circuit: bench press, squat, seated row, stepup, chinup, situp, shoulder press, and back extension. Complete two circuits, resting 2 minutes between them, and do 10 to 15 repetitions of each exercise.
Time: 18 minutes

2 CARDIO WORKOUT

Use this interval method. Start out at an easy pace (about 40 percent of your best effort) for 90 seconds. Then increase your speed to the fastest pace you can maintain (about 95 percent of your maximum) for 30 seconds. That's 1 interval. Repeat 5 times, for a total of 6 intervals.

It's short but intense, so it'll save you time. And unlike traditional steady-state aerobic exercise, it'll keep your body burning fat at a higher rate for hours after you've finished. You can perform it on the road or treadmill, but if you're packing more than an extra 20 pounds, opt for an exercise bike to reduce the stress on your knees.
Time: 12 minutes

Total: 30 minutes

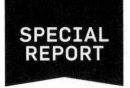
TAKE A WALK Research shows that the body prefers to use visceral fat for energy, says Dr. Ross. In a study that he published in the *Annals of Internal Medicine*, he and his team asked obese men to walk briskly or jog lightly every day for 3 months while eating enough to maintain their weight. The result: They reduced their visceral fat by 12 percent.

GO HARD Mild exercise whacks away at visceral fat, but strenuous activity has an even greater effect. Canadian researchers found that losing just 11 percent of your body weight can result in a 42 percent reduction in visceral fat; thus, a guy who weighs 205 pounds can cut his visceral fat in nearly half by losing 23 pounds. The best weight-loss plan: Cardio and strength training, each performed three times a week. Korean scientists found this formula to result in 4 more pounds of weight loss, and 11 percent more visceral fat loss, than cardio alone. (You'll find a plan that works exactly that magic when you read about the *Men's Health* Muscle System in Chapter 8.)

HOT TIP #52

Brew better health. Because of their high yeast content, wheat beers can actually help stabilize blood sugar and may even speed weight loss.

AND KEEP WORKING OUT Sumos consume up to 7,000 calories a day, but as long as they exercise—and their fat stores remain subcutaneous—their risks of heart disease and diabetes remain low. But if they stop exercising and continue eating heavily once they retire, their risk of diabetes shoots up. The lesson: Don't sweat the jiggles. Just sweat.

But keep in mind, that bulge around your middle isn't entirely your fault to begin with. The American food landscape, with the help of modern "food science," is conspiring to add to that repository of visceral fat. At every rest stop, gas station, airport, mall, and even gym, we are surrounded by food that really isn't food at all—it's mostly just varying concoctions of corn and soy mixed with sugar, all of which lead to weight gain if consumed in excess. And boy, do we consume them in excess.

CHILDREN OF THE CORN (AND SOY)

Practically every packaged-food product on the shelves at your local grocery store contains corn or soy. And when researchers from the University of Hawaii analyzed 480 servings of food (hamburgers, chicken sandwiches, and fries) from some of the most popular chain restaurants in the United States (McDonald's, Burger King, and Wendy's), they found that out of the 480 samples, only 12 burgers—bought at a Burger King on the West Coast—did not show traces of corn. Corn was present in the fat in the fries and in all chicken samples. And they didn't even bother to test the soft drinks, which are basically high-fructose corn syrup (HFCS) and food coloring, or the buns, which are sweetened with HFCS and chock-full of soy.

> **HOT TIP #53**
>
> **Don't diet drunk.** Booze can sabotage weight loss by whetting your appetite. People who drank alcohol before hitting a buffet ate 15 percent more, according to a recent British study. Save your drink for after dinner.

The problem with all of that corn and soy is that it means we're eating too much of what are called omega-6 fatty acids—fats that come from seeds like corn kernels and soybeans. (Heart-and-brain-healthy omega-3 fatty acids, on the other hand, come from things like seafood, leafy vegetables, and nuts.) And a disproportionately high level of omega-6 fatty acids—a family of fatty acids that compete with omega-3s for space in our cell membranes—promotes chronic inflammation, which leads to heart disease, cancer, Alzheimer's, and depression. Now, we need omega-6s in our diet. They're essential for heart and brain function. But, thanks to corn

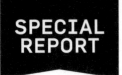

and soy, our foodscape has an omega-6 to omega-3 ratio of about 20:1. Ideally that ratio should be 1:1.

How did this get so out of whack? Just check any packaged-food label in your pantry, for starters. If a product contains "polyunsaturated fat," that's usually synonymous with omega-6 fatty acids. So are "high-fructose corn syrup" and "soy protein isolates." In fact, omega-6s have worked their way into virtually all 45,000 products at your local grocery.

And recent research indicates that an out-of-balance omega-6 to omega-3 ratio leads to adipogenesis—the creation of fat cells! In one study in the *British Journal of Nutrition*, mice fed a ratio of 6:1 (omega-6s to omega-3s) gained significantly more fat than mice on a 1:1.2 ratio. Another study, in the journal *Progress in Lipid Research,* determined that consuming more omega-6s than omega-3s leads to increased risk of fat development.

The consequences of this can be seen across the country, where 72 percent of the male population is overweight and 32 percent are obese. The consumption of HFCS alone, created by chemically altering cornmeal, has been linked to hormonal patterns that promote weight gain. Which is why, even if you've been dieting and exercising, you might not see the results you want. And you need to know that it's not your fault.

Now, your goal is not to get rid of omega-6s completely because they are essential to good health. But eating fewer packaged goods and more high-nutrition foods—and focusing on the *Men's Health* FAST & LEAN superfood groups—will help you cut your intake to more natural levels.

> **HOT TIP #54**
>
> **Get macho, eat some nachos.**
> Sometimes—like during the big game—you gotta eat junk. But if you work out beforehand, your muscles will sponge up large amounts of carbs, preventing fat storage.

HOW STRESS MAKES YOU FAT

1. STRESS HITS YOUR BRAIN

Hypothalamus: This gland in your brain responds to stress by secreting corticotropin-releasing hormone (CRH), which travels through the capillaries to the pituitary gland

Pituitary gland: Reacts to the CRH by releasing adrenocorticotropic hormone (ACTH)

Adrenal glands: Respond to the ACTH by flooding the bloodstream with two stress hormones, epinephrine (commonly called adrenaline) and cortisol

2. ADRENALINE

Adrenaline switches on the body's primordial fight-or-flight response:

- Heart rate and pulse quicken to send extra blood to the muscles and organs.
- Bronchial tubes dilate to accept extra oxygen to feed the brain and keep us alert.
- Blood vessels constrict to stem bleeding in case of an injury.

3. CORTISOL (YOUR FRIEND)

Cortisol and adrenaline release fat and sugar (glucose) into the bloodstream for use as energy to deal with the stressor in an emergency. That works perfectly during short-term stress, such as when you need to fend off the angry Rottweiler chasing your bike.

4. CORTISOL (YOUR ENEMY)

Cortisol can also signal your cells to store as much fat as possible and inhibit the body from releasing fat to burn as energy. This occurs when cortisol levels remain high due to long-term stressors, such as a lunatic boss, a pesky divorce attorney, or a teenager who insists on smoking dope in the living room. Chronically elevated cortisol disrupts the body's metabolic control systems: muscle breaks down, blood sugar rises, appetite increases, and you get fat! What's worse, the fat tends to accumulate in the abdominal region and on the artery walls, because visceral fat, which resides behind the abdominal muscles, has more cortisol receptors than does fat located just under the skin.

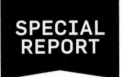

THE UNUSUAL SUSPECTS

Food manufacturers sneaking cheap corn and soy into everything from the hamburger bun to the hamburger itself is just one reason why your weight is not your fault. Here's a look at how stress, chemicals, hidden sugars, lack of sleep, and crafty food marketing are battling against your weight-loss efforts every day.

STRESS: Whether you're fending off an angry client, a disgruntled spouse, or heck, a charging sumo wrestler, your body's response to stress is the same: Your hypothalamus floods your blood with hormones to frighten you into action. Cortisol and epinephrine are your body's alarm-system hormones; they make your heart beat faster and dilate your bronchial tubes so they can feed oxygen to your brain to keep you alert. They also release fat and glucose into your bloodstream to provide emergency energy. But too much stress can keep your cortisol level consistently elevated, which disrupts your metabolic system. This, in turn, signals your cells to store as much fat as possible. Worse, the fat tends to accumulate in your belly as dangerous visceral fat, which resides behind your abdominal muscles and has more cortisol receptors than other fat does. (For a blow-by-blow account of this chemical process, see "How Stress Makes You Fat," on the previous page.)

> **HOT TIP #55**
>
> **Turn it up.** People could complete 10 additional reps when they listened to their favorite music while exercising, according to a College of Charleston study

FIGHT BACK: To defend yourself against stress-induced weight gain, make a habit of exercising 3 days a week, using the principles outlined in the *Men's Health* Muscle System. Doing so helps regulate your cortisol levels, say researchers at Ohio State University. Also try to eat organic foods as much as possible in order to steer clear of the common pesticide atrazine. A National Health and Environmental Effects Research Laboratory study showed that atrazine produced extreme increases in stress-hormone levels in rats. In fact, the stress reaction was similar to that seen when the animals were restrained against their will, the study noted.

ENDOCRINE-DISRUPTING CHEMICALS: There's a new threat to your belly—a class of natural and synthetic compounds known as endocrine-disrupting chemicals (EDCs), or as researchers have begun to call them, "obesogens." Obesogens are chemicals that disrupt the function of our endocrine systems, leading to weight gain and many of the diseases that curse the American populace. (The above-mentioned atrazine is one of them.) And because high school biology was probably a while back, here's a quick

> **HOT TIP #56**
>
> **Maximize minerals.** The bad breath might be worth it: Cooked onions and garlic help your body absorb more of certain key minerals such as iron and zinc from grains, according to a studying the *Journal of Agricultural and Food Chemistry.*

refresher: The endocrine system is made up of all the glands and cells that produce the hormones that regulate our bodies. Growth and development, sexual function, reproductive processes, mood, sleep, hunger, stress, metabolism, and the way our bodies use food—it's all controlled by hormones. But your endocrine system is a finely tuned instrument that can easily be thrown off-kilter. "Obesogens are thought to act by hijacking the regulatory systems that control body weight," said Frederick vom Saal, PhD, curators' professor of biological sciences at the University of Missouri. That's why endocrine disruptors are so good at making us fat—and that's why diet advice doesn't always work—because even strictly follow-

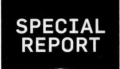

ing the smartest traditional advice won't lower your obesogen exposure. See, an apple a day may have kept the doctor away 250 years ago when Benjamin Franklin included the phrase in his almanac. But if that apple comes loaded with obesity-promoting chemicals—9 of the 10 most commonly used pesticides are obesogens, and apples are one of the most pesticide-laden foods out there—then Ben's advice is way out of date.

FIGHT BACK: Obesogens enter our bodies from a wide variety of sources—from natural hormones found in soy products, from artificial hormones fed to food animals, from plastic pollutants in some food packaging, from chemicals added to processed foods, and from pesticides sprayed on our produce. See "Your Guide to Avoiding Endocrine-Disrupting, Fat-Inducing Chemicals" at the end of this chapter for details on how to cleanse your body of these nasty fat-promoting invaders.

> **HOT TIP #57**
>
> **Go to Rio.** Just four Brazil nuts provide you with 100 percent of your RDA of selenium, a natural anxiety fighter.

HIDDEN SUGARS Eat a little sugar and you end up craving more, which means more calories and more girth. That's because sugar is addictive, seriously addictive. A group of Princeton University researchers found that eating sugar triggers the release of opioids, neurotransmitters that activate the brain's pleasure receptors. Addictive drugs, including morphine, target the same opioid receptors. That's right, sugar activates the same pathways that are stimulated by drugs such as heroin and morphine—which explains why we eat so much of it. According to a USDA survey, the average American eats about 20 teaspoons of added sugar daily, or 317 empty calories. Eighty-two percent of that added sugar is from soda, baked goods, breakfast cereals, candy, and fruit drinks. But sugar shows up in so many products, and under so many different names, that you may not even know you're eating it.

LOOK FOR THESE ALIASES: maltose, sorghum, sorbitol, dextrose, lactose, fructose, high fructose corn syrup, and glucose. And then there are the healthy-sounding versions: molasses, brown rice sugar, fruit juice, barley malt, honey, and organic cane juice.

FIGHT BACK: All sugars spike insulin levels and affect the body in the same way. A good rule is to skip any product that lists sugar as one of its first four ingredients. Doing this will help you to avoid fructose. New research from the University of California at San

DECODE ANY FOOD LABEL IN 4 EASY STEPS

Use this simple checklist to decode nutrition labels (and outwit marketers). Start with step one, and get rid of products from there.

1 NIX UNHEALTHY FATS: If a product contains partially hydrogenated or interesterified oils, you're eating trans fats, which have been linked to memory impairment, diabetes, and obesity. The term "stearate-rich" means essentially the same thing.

2 LIMIT SUGARS: Always choose the food with the least amount. If a product has more than 8 grams per serving, put it back.

3 CHOOSE FIBER: The more, the better, as fiber slows digestion and helps prevent the spikes in blood sugar that lead to obesity and insulin resistance. Buyer beware: Sneaky manufacturers often add isolated fibers such as inulin and maltodextrin to foods so they can make fiber claims on their packaging, but these are no substitute for whole grains.

4 COUNT INGREDIENTS: Choose the item that has the closest to one.

Francisco (UCSF) indicates that fructose (our greatest source of which is high-fructose corn syrup, which the average American consumes at a rate of 12 teaspoons a day) can trick your brain into craving more food, even when you're full. And preliminary research indicates that fructose may even play a role in disrupting our endocrine systems, by interfering with our ability to process leptin, the hormone that tells us when we're full, said Robert Lustig, MD, a pediatric endocrinologist at UCSF. But it's not just HFCS and table syrup that you need to avoid; fruit juice can be as bad as soda. In fact, 100 percent fruit juice has 1.8 grams of fructose per ounce, while soda has 1.7 grams per ounce.

SLEEPLESSNESS: A sleep schedule is vital to any weight-loss plan. Too much or too little shut-eye can add extra pounds. In a new study, Canadian scientists revealed that sleeping for 5 to 6 hours a night makes you 69 percent more likely to pack on pounds than if you log 8 hours. What's just as surprising is that snoozing for 9 to 10 hours also increases your risk of becoming overweight by 38 percent. "Lack of sleep releases hormones that stimulate your appetite," said study author Jean-Philippe Chaput, PhD. "But oversleeping means you'll burn less energy in a day, since you aren't as active." Plus, an Australian study found that dozing late on weekends leaves you more tired on Monday and Tuesday, compared with sticking to your work wake-up time. People with sleep deficits tend to eat more (and use less energy) because they're tired, according to Wake Forest University researchers, while those who sleep longer than 8 hours a night may be less active.

> **HOT TIP #58**
>
> **Don't patrol the border.** The average margarita has 3 times as many calories as a Cosmopolitan and 4½ times as many as a glass of wine.

FIGHT BACK: Make sure you have good melatonin rhythm. When the sun goes down, your pineal gland switches on like clockwork to secrete melatonin, a hormone that helps you fall asleep and regulates your circadian rhythm. It lowers your core body temperature, which if too high promotes wakefulness. Production of melatonin peaks in the middle of the night, and the process can be disrupted by even very low levels of artificial light. Darkness is the key to good melatonin rhythm. Buy heavy curtains, cover your alarm clock, and turn off gadgets. Make it dark enough that you can't see your hand. If you go to the bathroom and turn on that bright light, you'll lower melatonin almost immediately. So use a red night-light (or heat lamp) in your bathroom, because red light has less effect on melatonin than white or blue light.

> **HOT TIP #59**
>
> **Eat a better butter.** Almond butter has more calcium and magnesium, 60 percent more healthy fat, and three times as much vitamin E as peanut butter.

SNEAKY SUPERMARKET TRICKS: Food manufacturers think you're stupid. And their marketing strategies rely on it. For instance, the makers of Swedish Fish, Mike and Ike, and Good & Plenty may be hoping you'll equate the "fat-free" label they have plastered on their candy boxes with "healthy" or "nonfattening" so you'll forget about all the sugar their products contain. It's a distraction device: Food companies advertise what they want you to notice—and the candy aisle is just the start. They can also get away with marking their calorie counts in a misleading way—for example, by declaring that bottle of juice to be 2½ servings, when clearly you're meant to drink the whole thing. Many of the packaged-food offenders are obvious—you already know that double-cheese-and-pepperoni calzones are a health hazard—but a lot of the worst products are double agents.

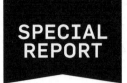
They pose as healthy choices, labeled with such comforting words as "fortified," "lite," "all natural," and even "multi-grain." But these words are meaningless in reality.

FIGHT BACK: Think of the grocery store as a battleground, and the edges of the store—where produce, dairy products, and meat are sold—as your green zone. Stay there, and make only strategic, solo incursions into the middle aisles to snag beans and whole-grain cereals. But be aware: A label that says "made with whole grain" doesn't necessarily mean it's healthy. Pick up a box of General Mills Franken Berry and you'll see what we mean. A product needs to be made of only 51 percent whole-grain flour in order to carry this label. To make sure you're getting a truly whole-grain product, check that the word "whole" is next to every flour listed. And know that the newest marketing ploy, describing foods as "all natural," has no specific government standards, and there's no legislation in the works for it. Just about anything can be called "all natural."

> **HOT TIP #60**
>
> **Stand up for your health.**
> Your core works 20 percent harder when performing a standing cable chest press than during a standard barbell bench press.

YOUR GUIDE TO AVOIDING ENDOCRINE-DISRUPTING, FAT-INDUCING CHEMICALS

Our foods, even foods we consider "health" or "diet" foods, are loaded with endocrine-disrupting chemicals (EDSs) that prime your body for fat storage. Here's what you need to do to avoid them.

KNOW WHEN TO GO ORGANIC

The average American is exposed to 10 to 13 different pesticides through food, beverages, and drinking water every day, and 9 of the 10 most common pesticdes are EDCs. But according to a recent study in the journal Environmental Health Perspectives, eating an organic diet for just 5 days can reduce circulating pesticide EDCs to undetectable or near undetectable levels. Of course, organic foods can be expensive. But going 100 percent organic isn't necessary—many foods have such low levels of pesticides that buying organic just isn't worth it. The Environmental Working Group (EWG) calculated that you can reduce your pesticide exposure by nearly 80 percent simply by choosing organic for the 12 fruits and vegetables shown in their tests to contain the highest levels of pesticides. They call them "The Dirty Dozen," and (starting with the worst) they are celery, peaches, strawberries, apples, blueberries (domestic), nectarines, bell peppers, spinach, kale/collard greens, cherries, potatoes, and grapes (imported). And you can feel good about buying the following 15 conventionally grown fruits and vegetables that the EWG dubbed "The Clean Fifteen," because they were shown to have little pesticide residue: onions, avocados, sweet corn (frozen), pineapples, mangoes, sweet peas (frozen), asparagus, kiwifruits, cabbage, eggplant, cantaloupe (domestic), watermelons, grapefruits, sweet potatoes, and honeydew melons.

DON'T EAT PLASTIC

You're probably thinking, "Well, I don't generally eat plastic." Ah, but you do. Chances are that you're among the 93 percent of Americans with detectable levels of bisphenol-A (BPA) in their bodies and that you're also among the 75 percent of Americans with detectable levels of phthalates. Both are synthetic chemicals that mimic estrogen—essentially, artificial female hormones—and they leach into our foods from plastic or aluminum food packaging. These plastic-based chemicals trick our bodies into storing fat and not building or retaining muscle. Decreasing your exposure to plastic-based obesogens will maximize your chances both of losing unwanted flab and of building lean muscle mass. Here's how:

1. Never heat food in plastic containers or put plastic items in the dishwasher, which can increase the amount of BPA they release. BPA leaches from polycarbonate sports bottles 55 times faster when exposed to boiling liquids as opposed to cold ones, according to a study in the journal *Toxicology Letters*.

2. Avoid buying fatty foods like meats that are packaged in plastic wrap, because EDCs are stored in fatty tissue. The plastic wrap used at the supermarket is mostly PVC, whereas the plastic wrap you buy to wrap things at home is increasingly made from more benign polyethylene.

3. Cut down on canned goods; choose food like tuna in a pouch instead of a can.

GO LEAN

Whenever possible, choose pasture-raised meats, which, studies show, have less fat than their confined, grain-fed counterparts and none of the weight-promoting hormones. Plus, grass-fed beef contains 60 percent more omega-3s, 200 percent more vitamin E, and two to three times more conjugated linoleic acid (CLA, a nutrient that helps ward off heart disease, cancer, and diabetes and can help you lose weight, according to a study in the *American Journal of Clinical Nutrition*) than conventionally raised beef. And select sustainable lean fish with low levels of toxins like mercury and PCBs. A study in the journal *Occupational and Environmental Medicine* found that even though the pesticide DDT was banned in 1973, the chemical and its breakdown product, DDE, can still be found today in fatty fish. Bigger fish eat smaller fish and so carry a much higher toxic load. Avoid ahi or bigeye tuna, tilefish, swordfish, shark, and marlin. Focus on smaller fish like anchovies, and mackerel and wild-caught Alaskan salmon. Choose farmed rainbow trout, farmed mussels, scallops (bay, farmed), Pacific halibut, tuna, and mahimahi. When you cook fish, broil, grill, or bake it instead of pan-frying—this will allow contaminants from the fatty portions of fish to drain out.

FILTER YOUR WATER

The best way to eliminate EDCs from your tap water is an activated carbon water filter. Available for faucets and pitchers and as under-the-sink units, these filters remove most pesticides and industrial pollutants. Check the label to make sure the filter meets the National Science Foundation/American National Standards Institute's standard 53, indicating that it treats water for both health and aesthetic concerns.

The rounder and harder your belly, the more it puts your health in danger.

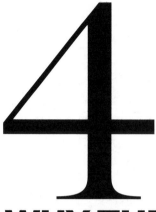

WHY THE SMARTEST DIET IS NO DIET AT ALL

HOW TO TURN FAT INTO MUSCLE WITHOUT GIVING UP ANYTHING, EVER (SERIOUSLY).

By this stage in our story, you've already learned a lot about fitness, nutrition, and weight loss. You've taken a quick quiz that helped you measure your fitness level, and you've picked up plenty of cool tips on looking and feeling your best. Now you're ready to head into a bold new future—with a bold new body. But before we charge forward, let's see what you've learned so far. Answer this question, and you'll be ready to move on to our next round.

You are most likely headed for a future of obesity if:

A. The last athletic award you won was a Pabst Blue Ribbon
B. The street address on your driver's license is "Kirstie Alley"
C. You think the term "fruit and nut bar" refers to the joint where you met your ex-wife
D. You are currently, right now, at this very moment, on a diet

And the answer is: D!

(Actually, the answer is B, but that's not really relevant for most of you dudes.)

It seems counterintuitive, but studies have shown time and again that the biggest predictor of your being overweight in the future is whether or not you're on a diet right now. Indeed, almost every diet plan out there is designed to make you gain pounds in the long term.

Wow. Really? WTF?

So why did we have you shell out big bucks for this *Men's Health Diet* book when there are so many lonely women down at the local gin joint who could use a wine spritzer or two?

Well, first off, we said *almost* every diet plan out there will make you gain flab. The *Men's Health* Nutrition System is a different animal entirely. But before we explain how, let us tell you . . .

The Trouble with Traditional Diets

There are tens of thousands of diet plans out there, touted by doctors, by celebrities, by athletes, by whatever Richard Simmons is—all sorts of schemes, some sensible and most pretty crazy. And every single one of them has one thing in common:

They all work. Kind of. Sort of. For a little while.

You see, every diet plan works to a certain degree, because every diet you go on forces you to pay attention to the food you eat—and that alone helps cut down on your calorie intake. Who cares if some of those schemes sound a little wacky—grapefruit diets, cabbage soup diets, cottage cheese diets, mayonnaise-and-Slim Jim diets? (Okay, I made that last one up.) And who cares if the natural act of eating becomes an exercise in trigonometry as you try to calculate your calorie intake and phases and "pods" and ratios and points and all the other bizarre mathematical formulas out there? The good news for the nearly 76 million Americans who are on a diet of some kind at this very moment is that, in the short term, every single one of them will work.

And the bad news? In the long term, said UCLA researchers, two-thirds of people who lose weight on a diet plan end up weighing more a year or two later than when they started! Heck, diets are the Florida condo markets of health and fitness.

So how do you know if a diet is destined to fail? The same way you tell if a car or a quarterback or a real estate market is going to break down: You run it through a series of tests. Here, then, is the three-point *Men's Health* Diet Diagnostic.

> **HOT TIP #61**
>
> **Get a milk mustache.** Consuming 1,800 milligrams of calcium a day could block the absorption of about 80 calories, according to a University of Tennessee study. Jump-start your intake by filling your coffee mug with milk, drinking it down to the level you want in your coffee, then pouring in the java. That's 300 milligrams!

TROUBLE SIGN #1: You have to eliminate an entire food group. When a diet calls itself "low fat" or "high carb," or has a period where you "cleanse" your body with shakes and smoothies, that's not weight-loss magic, that's calorie restriction. A recent study in the *New England Journal of Medicine* found that regardless of the type of diet you choose—whether it bans carbs or fats or sodium or meat or cheese or, heck, frittatas and fruitcakes—it will lead to weight loss, because banning a particular food group will automatically create a calorie deficit. This finding is echoed in other recent studies published in the journals *Diabetes Care*, the *American Journal of Clinical Nutrition*, and the *Archives of Internal Medicine*. But the thing about calorie restriction is that it isn't sustainable, it can actually be harmful (especially if you're concerned about building and maintaining lean muscle), and it leads to weight gain down the road.

> **HOT TIP #62**
>
> **Skip the sodas.** Chugging two or more sodas a week could raise your risk of pancreatic cancer by 87 percent, according to a study published in *Cancer Epidemiology, Biomarkers & Prevention*.

Recently, scientists reporting in the journal *Psychosomatic Medicine* investigated how the body reacts when you: (a) monitor your caloric intake, or (b) restrict your caloric intake. They found that restricting calories increases circulating levels of the stress hormone cortisol and that simply monitoring calories increases perceived stress. (Cortisol is a stress hormone that tells your body trouble's brewing and basically forces you to store calories as flab to prepare for hard times.) They concluded that "dieting, or the restriction of caloric intake, is ineffective because it increases chronic psychological stress and cortisol production—two factors that are known to cause weight gain." The study authors added that dieting in general may be be harmful to your psychological as well as physical well-being. (That's why the *Men's Health* Diet is all about eating more, not eating less.)

TROUBLE SIGN #2: You have to follow a formula, algorithm, or strict calorie allotment point-tallying system to figure out what to eat.

Cognitive scientists from Indiana University and the Max Planck Institute for Human Development in Berlin discovered recently that the more complex a diet appears to be, the more likely you are to quit it. The study authors compared the results of women following either the Weight Watchers point system or a simple diet that recommended specific foods and meals. They found that simply perceiving that your diet plan is complex (regardless of how simple it might actually be) makes it 54 percent more likely that you will prematurely give up said diet. (That's why I made the *Men's Health* Diet so simple—all you need to do is eyeball your portions, as outlined in Chapter 6.)

TROUBLE SIGN #3: You're told that if you base your diet on one single nutrient or food, you'll lose weight. You've seen them advertised: The Apple Diet. The Apple Cider Vinegar Diet. The Pineapple Diet. (And those are just a few that include the word "apple"!) These strange fad diets are two things: (1) calorie restriction in disguise, and (2) deprivation diets that don't let you enjoy the full bounty of nutrition that nature has to offer. For both of these reasons, diets like this are unsustainable and will ultimately lead to rebound weight gain. We simply can't exist on a narrow spectrum of food. Our taste buds crave diversity, and for good reason: A varied diet is a healthy diet. So, when we deny ourselves nutrition for the sake of weight loss, our bodies rebel.

> **HOT TIP #63**
>
> **Block blisters.**
> For long workouts, spread a little bit of Vaseline on the bottom of your feet and in between your toes. This will keep sweaty feet from blistering.

A study published in the *International Journal of Obesity* found that 91 percent of people going on a diet experience food cravings; once you start restricting calories, that figure goes up to 94 percent. And—this is the really creepy part—every time you resist a piece of

pie or a bagel with cream cheese or whatever your favorite indulgence is, you decrease your chances of being able to do it again.
That's because the ability to control ourselves wanes after we first
exert self-control, according to a new study from Florida State University. The reason? Self-control is fueled by ... wait for it ... sugar. Glucose to be exact. So every time you say no to those carbs, you increase your need for the very nutrients they contain. Ouch!

Indeed, most popular diets are just variations on the three themes discussed above. Let's take a tour through some of the top weight-loss plans out there and see if anything looks familiar.

The Zone Diet

The guiding principle of this particular diet is that high insulin levels contribute to weight gain—therefore, stabilizing insulin leads to weight loss. Okay, sounds reasonable. But, to accomplish this goal, every meal has to have a specific ratio of carbs, protein, and fat: 40 percent carbs, 30 percent protein, and 30 per-cent fat. That's the "zone" you need to be in all the time. You eat low-fat proteins at every meal; focus on good fats like the monoun-saturated fat in olive oil, almonds, and avocados and the omega-3 fatty acids in fish; limit carb intake to whole grains and some fruits while avoiding fruit juices, beer, and sweets; restrict saturated fat from red meat and egg yolks; and avoid processed foods ... Whew.

And that's just the basic diet. Foods are grouped into "blocks" based on their protein, fat, and carb content so one block of food will deliver the magical 40-30-30 ratio. You are allotted so many

> **HOT TIP #64**
>
> **Ruin your appetite.**
> Consuming a liquid —whether it's two glasses of water or a cup of soup— to begin a meal can fill you up and reduce your total calorie intake by up to 20 percent. Try this: Drink one glass of H_2O and have a broth-based soup, like miso, minestrone, or chicken noodle, as an appetizer.

blocks a day depending on how much you exercise.

Now, The Zone gets credit for trying to balance essential nutrients while attempting not to restrict too many foods. But, according to a recent study in the *Journal of the American Medical Association*, the diet has the same effect on insulin levels as all the other popular diets. So basically all of that counting of carbs, proteins, and fats to make sure they're proportioned right for each meal does little more than make you hyperaware of the foods you're eating, which can help you cut back on calories and lose weight.

And did you recognize one or more of the trouble signs from the *Men's Health* Diet Diagnostics? Yep, rule number two stands out: This diet is way too complex and therefore is probably unsustainable. Now, to be fair, the plan does offer prepackaged foods that fit its formula, but they're highly processed and seriously unnatural—in fact, some of these "food" products were among the many diet aids that were recalled by their manufacturer in 2009 for containing tainted peanut butter.

The Atkins Diet

It's a low-carbohydrate, high-fat diet consisting of four phases. Phase 1 eliminates almost all carbohydrates: You're allowed only 20 grams a day, which means no bread, pasta, fruits, vegetables, or juices, just proteins and fats. Phase 2 increases carbohydrate intake to 25 grams a day for a week, and each week thereafter you increase your carb intake by 5 grams. You continue like this until you stop losing weight, at which time you decrease your carb intake by 5 grams daily to reinitiate weight loss (that's Phase 3). Phase 4 is based on the number of grams of carbs you need to maintain your weight. I don't know about you, but

> **HOT TIP #65**
>
> **Hold for muscles.** Simply holding barbells or dumbbells strengthens your wrists and forearms by as much as 25 percent and 16 percent, respectively, in 12 weeks, according to a study at Auburn University.

aside from needing a cookie every now and again, going without fruits and vegetables—the very foods that study after study says are key to health and longevity—seems counterproductive.

The diet's emphasis on protein is on the right track—a recent study in the *American Journal of Clinical Nutrition* found that while a calorie deficit is the main factor in weight loss, those who get 30 percent of their daily calories from protein feel more satiated than those who eat less protein, leading them to consume 441 fewer calories a day and lose 5 pounds over 2 weeks. But Atkins takes this idea to the extreme. And in reality it's just camouflaged calorie restriction. Of course you're going to lose weight if you restrict a nutrient group completely! You're dramatically decreasing the number of calories you're putting in your body. But you're also losing out on a whole spectrum of wonderful tastes, smells, and textures that your body craves. This diet is guilty of all three trouble signs!

HOT TIP #66

Rebuff rejection. For a broken heart, try Tylenol. In a new study in *Psychological Science*, people who took 1,000 milligrams of acetaminophen daily for 3 weeks felt gradual relief from the sting of social rejection. The reason: Acetaminophen raises your brain's threshold for both physical and emotional pain.

Which means it's just not sustainable. Restricting foods will only make you crave them more, and you may end up bingeing instead. The bottom line is that you might lose weight to begin with, but keeping it off is another story.

Weight Watchers

Here, every serving of food has a value based on its calorie, fat, and fiber content. Greater amounts of fiber decrease the point value assigned to a particular food, whereas more fat and calories increase the point value. Your job is to stay under a certain number of points every day in order to achieve your weight-loss goals. You can choose between a high-carb and high-protein plan.

Now, the folks at Weight Watchers deserve credit for helping people realize how many calories they're putting into their bodies. And they're really focused on providing social support, an important aspect of weight management. But while monitoring your daily calorie intake is a great exercise for those who want to lose weight, ultimately it is just that, an exercise. Counting calories is not something you want to do for the rest of your life. Food is meant to be enjoyed, after all. On top of that, the point system can have the unintended effect of slowing your metabolism if, say, you eat all of your points in one meal and then starve yourself for the rest of the day (more on that in an upcoming chapter). This diet is the poster child for trouble sign number two.

THE BOTTOM LINE FOR ALL OF THESE DIETS, AND MANY OTHERS OUT THERE, IS THIS: Gimmicks don't work. We're surrounded by food all of the time, some of it healthy, some not so much. But no point system is going to help you navigate the food terrain you're confronted with every day. And depriving yourself of the foods you crave can only last so long before it comes back to bite you. The *Men's Health* Nutrition System takes into account your whole food landscape and offers you a diet—no, a lifestyle—that allows you to eat the foods you love and helps you shed pounds and keep them off.

5

HOW TO TRICK YOUR BODY INTO BURNING FAT
MEET YOUR BEST DEFENSE AGAINST WEIGHT GAIN: MORE MUSCLE.

How would you like to magically burn off about 40 calories in the next 15 minutes without even breaking a sweat? Want to try? Okay, here's what you do:

Go into the bedroom. Open up the closet. Look inside. Anything need to go to the dry cleaners? What about that blazer with the chicken wing sauce on it? Okay, toss it in a bag. Straighten a few other hanging items, and fold your sweatshirts so the inside of your wardrobe doesn't look like you had to flee the Sopranos really fast. Good job. Now have a seat.

Presto! You've just smoked 40 or more calories in less time than it takes Snoop Dogg to burn a blunt, and all you did was neaten up your clothes. Magic, right?

Well, not really. You see, your body is already primed to be a fat-burning machine. All you need to do to start changing your body's shape is tune up that fat furnace and get it revving at maximum efficiency so you'll burning even more fat while going about the mundane rituals of life.

> **HOT TIP #67**
>
> **Seed for the future.** Pumpkin seeds are the easiest way to consume more magnesium, which French researchers have linked to longevity.

This fat-burning magic is performed by your metabolism, a word you've probably heard tossed around a lot but maybe don't quite understand. What is metabolism? Simply put, it's all of the various chemical reactions that happen inside your body 24-7 to keep you alive. It's food being turned into energy and that energy being burned to keep your hair growing, your heart beating, your liver pumping out bile, your lungs transferring oxygen to your blood cells, and your kidneys turning Coors Light into urine (not that there's a huge leap there). It's the engine room of your individual starship, your never-ending calorie burn. And while you may imagine that the majority of your calories get burned while you're engaged in some strenuous activity like riding a bike, diving into a pool, or doing the parallel polka with a pulchritudinous partner, you'll actually burn most of your calories, well, just keeping the lights on.

In fact, think of metabolism as your caloric 401(k) program. It's not going to give you instant gratification, like throwing down a week's pay on black and letting it ride. It's a long-term strategy, but it's a sure thing: Invest in it, and you'll get slow, steady, effective returns that will keep you happy and healthy for years to come.

Now, like any long-term investment, your body's engine needs a little maintenance from time to time. In this chapter, I'll show you the smart ways to tweak your metabolism, improving your burn just enough so you use up more and more calories over the long haul. (Or as they say in financial circles, it's time to work less for your calorie burn, and have your calorie burn start working for you!) Prepare for a few surprises, starting with . . .

Why Burning Calories in the Gym Is a Waste of Time

Whoa—did that just say what you thought it said? That burning calories in the gym is "a waste of time"? Is this a *Men's Health* book, or did I slip Lewis Black's autobiography between the covers?

Well, stay with me. Burning calories in the gym is great—in fact, in Chapter 8, you'll learn about the *Men's Health* Muscle System, our most effective fat-burning plan ever, designed to burn 160-plus calories off a 180-pound man in just 15 minutes. But the energy you exhaust while you're in the gym isn't as big a deal as those tired old LED readouts on the treadmill might make it seem. See, we all have three "burns" that make up our metabolism:

BURN #1: Basal (resting) metabolism. Your basal metabolic rate (BMR) accounts for 60 to 70 percent of your overall metabolism, and surprisingly, it's the number of calories you burn doing nothing at all: lying in bed staring at the ceiling or veggin' on the couch watching TV. As I said above, it is fueled by the inner workings of your body— your heart beating, your lungs breathing, even your cells dividing.

BURN #2: Digestive metabolism, or the thermic effect of food (TEF). Simply digesting food—turning carbs into sugar and protein into amino acids—typically burns 10 to 15 percent of your daily calories. Protein burns more calories during digestion than carbohydrates and fat, about 25 calories for every 100 calories consumed. Carbohydrates and fat burn 10 to 15 calories for every 100 consumed. (You'll see why this is important to remember in a future chapter.)

So pause a moment to think about this: Between 70 and 85 percent of the calories you burn every day go to either eating or just hanging around doing nothing.

So, what about the other 15 to 30 percent?

BURN #3: Exercise and movement metabolism. This part of your metabolism includes both workouts at the gym and other, more enjoyable physical activities (it's called "exercise-activity thermogenesis," or EAT) and countless incidental movements throughout the day, like turning the pages of this book and twiddling your thumbs (that's called "non-exercise-activity thermogenesis," or NEAT).

So, here's an interesting question: Why is it so hard to lose weight just by exercising? Why are there so many fat people in the gym? The answer is simple. Exercise and movement account for only 15 to 30 percent of your fat burn. Up to 85 percent of the calories you burn in a given day have nothing to do with moving your body!

So, skip the gym, right? Not quite. Because exercise plays an important role in preparing your body to burn off your great health threat: belly fat.

Why the Fatter You Get, the Fatter You'll Get

Fat doesn't just show up at your door one day, rent a room, and live quietly alone with a couple of cats. Fat loves company. Fat's building a cocktail party crowd that never goes home, and the center of conversation is right beneath your belly button. The more fat you open the door to, the harder it will be to stop even more fat from inviting itself to your potbelly Promised Land. Here's why.

Your BMR, or resting metabolic rate—which eats up the majority of your daily calorie burn—is determined by two things: your mom and dad, and the amount of fat versus muscle in your body. And while you can't change who your parents are (if you could, there would be no children on *Real Housewives of New Jersey*), you can improve the other part of the equation and turn your resting metabolism up a few notches.

Problem is, fat plays its own role in the metabolic game, and it's literally working to slow down your calorie burn. "Fat and lazy" is a pretty accurate description from a scientific standpoint. Fat is lazy on a metabolic level. It burns barely any calories at all. For your body to support a pound of fat, it needs to burn up a mere 2 calories a day. Muscle, on the other hand, is very metabolically active. At rest, 1 pound of muscle burns three times as many calories every day just to sustain itself—and a lot of those calories that muscle burns off come from fat storage units. That's why fat hates muscle, because muscle is constantly burning it off.

> **HOT TIP #68**
>
> **Get juiced for sleep.** Cherry juice is a concentrated source of melatonin, an effective sleep aid. Just beware of juice blends with high levels of sugar.

So fat actually fights back, trying to erode muscle so it can get more of its fat friends into your body. The real bad guy in this internal battle that's happening right now in your body is a nasty character called "visceral fat." As you read in our Special Report, visceral fat is the kind that resides behind the abdominal muscles, surrounding your internal organs (the viscera). And visceral fat works its mischief by releasing a number of substances collectively called adipokines. Adipokines include compounds that raise your risks of high blood pressure, diabetes, inflammation, and heart disease. Visceral fat also messes with an important hormone called adiponectin, which regulates metabolism. The more visceral fat you have, the less adiponectin you have and the lower your metabolism. So fat literally begets more fat.

A study published in the *Journal of Applied Physiology* showed that those biologically active molecules that are released from visceral fat can actually degrade muscle quality—which, again, leads to more fat. The solution?

BURN, BABY, BURN

Calories burned per hour by a 180-pound man

1.	SITTING AT A DESK	**147**
2.	HAVING SEX	**160**
3.	PLAYING VOLLEYBALL	**327**
4.	CANOEING	**368**
5.	GOLFING	**368**
6.	KAYAKING	**409**
7.	HIKING	**491**
8.	SURFING	**518**
9.	PLAYING TENNIS	**573**
10.	DOING BODY-WEIGHT CALISTHENICS IN THE SAND	**286–655**
11.	SWIMMING	**573**
12.	STRENGTH TRAINING	**655**
13.	PLAYING BASKETBALL	**655**
14.	PLAYING ULTIMATE FRISBEE	**655**
15.	ROAD RUNNING	**655**
16.	MOUNTAIN BIKING ON HILLY TERRAIN	**695**
17.	TRAIL RUNNING HILLS	**736**
18.	RUNNING IN SAND	**769**
19.	PLAYING SOCCER	**573–818**
20.	CYCLING VIGOROUSLY UPHILL	**655–818**
21.	BOULDERING	**900**
22.	ROWING	**573–982**
23.	RUNNING UP STAIRS	**1,221**

Source: *Compendium of Physical Activities Tracking Guide*

More muscle.

After age 25, we all start to lose muscle mass if we don't do any-thing to stop the decline: ⅕ of a pound of muscle a year from ages 25 to 50, and then up to a pound of muscle a year. On top of a slump-ing metabolic rate, loss of muscle strength and mass are empiri-cally linked to a weaker immune system, not to mention weaker bones, stiffer joints, and slumping. Muscle mass has also been shown to play a central role in the response to stress. Further research is expected to show measurable links between diminished muscle mass and cancer mortality.

Muscle mass also plays a key role in preventing more common, but no less deadly, conditions such as cardiovascular disease and dia-betes. A survey of scientific literature published in the journal *Circu-lation* in 2006 linked the loss of muscle mass to insulin resistance (the main factor in type 2 diabetes), elevated lipid levels in the blood, and increased body fat, especially visceral fat.

See? It's a war. And if you want to stop the bad guy—visceral fat—you need to call in more reinforcements.

Why the Most Important Calories You Can Burn Are the Ones You're Burning Right Now

As you've learned, muscle is your body's defense against the onslaught of fat. That's why the *Men's Health* Muscle System is the perfect arma-ment upgrade. It's a simple weight-training regimen with an aerobic edge that will help your body attack fat even while you're at rest. It works in three simple ways, for three simple reasons:

First, as I said earlier, a pound of flab burns only 2 calories a day, while the same amount of muscle burns an estimated 6 calories a day, researchers believe. ("Many factors are at play, so call this the best educated guess," says Jeff Volek, PhD, RD, exercise and nutrition expert at the University of Connecticut.) So the more muscle you have, the more fat you burn, all day every day. That's why the *Men's Health* Muscle System focuses on adding lean muscle to your physique.

Second, while muscle burns calories, new muscle burns more calories. That's because the physical work you need to do to build and maintain new muscle can have a dramatic effect on your overall metabolism. Research shows that a single weight-training session can spike your calorie burn for up to 39 hours after you lift. (And remember, this doesn't include the calories you'll be burning off while you're actually exercising—more than 10 calories a minute, or 655 an hour. Think of those as just a bonus.)

And the long-term calorie burn you get from weight training doesn't just get rid of extra weight. It specifically targets belly fat! In a study conducted by Volek, overweight people following a reduced-calorie diet were divided into three groups. One group

MEASURE YOUR METABOLIC RATE

The best way to measure your daily calorie burn is to look honestly at the amount of calories you consume in a day. You can do this with a food log containing a full list of all the foods and liquids you ingest daily for a minimum of 3 days. (Try the USDA's online tool at mypyramidtracker.gov.) If you're not gaining weight, then your daily calorie consumption is also your daily metabolic rate. If you're packing on the pounds, your metabolic rate is lower than your calorie intake, and you need to tweak your eating habits.

If foods logs aren't for you, gyms and health clubs usually have devices you can use to assess your metabolic rate. The Bod Pod, for example, has pressure sensors that measure the air your body displaces when you sit in it. The machine uses that information to determine your muscle-to-fat ratio (to find one near you, go to bodpod.com).

didn't exercise, another performed aerobic exercise three days a week, and a third group did both aerobics and weight training three days a week. The results: Each group lost about the same amount of weight—21 pounds on average per person in 12 weeks. But those who lifted weights shed 5 pounds more fat than those who didn't pump iron. The weight they lost was almost pure fat, while the other two groups shed 15 pounds of lard *but also 5-plus pounds of muscle.* "Think about that," says Volek. "For the same amount of exercise time, with diets being equal, the participants who lifted lost almost 40 percent more fat."

> **HOT TIP #69**
>
> **Stagger yourself.** The next time you do pushups, stagger your hands—it'll increase the challenge to your core and shoulder muscles.

And the third, even more exciting reason why weight training is the ultimate fat fighter: The more muscle you have, the better your body's ability to use the nutrients you eat and the less likely it is to store your food (even junk food) as fat.

See, your muscles store energy (read: calories) in the form of glycogen. When you exercise, your muscles have to call on that glycogen to perform the work they're being tasked with doing. (When you get that weak-kneed feeling at the end of a footrace, that's your leg muscles telling you their glycogen tank is hitting zero.) One of the (many) advantages to working out is that after you exercise, your fat-storing hormones are subdued because your body wants to use incoming carbohydrates to restore the glycogen that was depleted during your workout. So the carbs you eat after exercise get stored in your muscles, not in your spare tire.

But it gets better: Your body—which is still burning calories at an advanced rate hours after your workout finishes—is now desperate to come up with energy to keep your brain thinking and your heart beating and your fingernails growing. And since all the food you're eating is being stored in your muscles, your body has to start hunting around for something else to burn.

Oh, here's something I can burn: belly fat!

And because aerobic exercise calls on glycogen too, incorporating a bit of aerobic exercise into your weight routine can enhance that effect. A study in the *British Journal of Nutrition* found that after 90 minutes of moderate-intensity cycling, a postexercise meal of nearly a pound of pasta (400 grams of cooked pasta yielding 297 grams of carbs) resulted in zero fat creation.

HOT TIP #70

Eat melons, skip melanoma. One slice of watermelon contains up to 10 milligrams of cancer-fighting lycopene—as much as four tomatoes.

You read that right—a pound of pasta and no fat creation. All of those carbs were shuttled back into the muscles for later use. That's why the *Men's Health* Muscle System keeps you working quickly and efficiently, creating an aerobic burn even as you build muscle. (That, and because you're a busy guy.)

And the extra benefit to the *Men's Health* Muscle System: You get to indulge in your favorite foods. In fact, what you eat after your workout can be your most indulgent meal of the day. You can eat more calories and even enjoy a little something sweet after your workout: Research shows that a combination of carbohydrates (some from sugar) and protein is the best concoction for speeding muscle growth. A superfast, supercheap answer: chocolate milk. Sure, there are plenty of expensive muscle shakes for sale at your gym, but more than five research universities have concluded that the stuff you drank in fourth grade remains the ultimate biceps-building cocktail.

HOW TO LOSE
21 POUNDS THIS YEAR
WITHOUT CHANGING ANYTHING

CONSIDER THIS: For every 10 additional calories you burn a day, you'll lose a pound a year. So if you could burn off a mere 210 more calories a day, you could lose 21 pounds. And you could do that without ever stepping foot in a gym. You just need to tweak your everyday routine.

CASE IN POINT: the five simple strategies below. Infuse them into your life, and you can instantly—and almost effortlessly—burn about 10 percent more calories a day.

+	**+**	**+**	**+**	**+**
DO THIS	**DO THIS**	**DO THIS**	**DO THIS**	**DO THIS**
Go for a brisk 20-minute walk	Stand during three 10-minute phone calls	Play vigorously with your kids or pet for 15 minutes	Spend 15 minutes washing the dishes	Take 10 minutes to straighten up one room
−	**−**	**−**	**−**	**−**
NOT THIS	**NOT THIS**	**NOT THIS**	**NOT THIS**	**NOT THIS**
Sit for your entire lunch hour	Put your feet up on your desk	Watch TV before dinner	Head straight to the couch	Go right to bed after dinner
=	**=**	**=**	**=**	**=**
EQUALS	**EQUALS**	**EQUALS**	**EQUALS**	**EQUALS**
49 extra calories burned	33 extra calories burned	82 extra calories burned	27 extra calories burned	21 extra calories burned

212 TOTAL EXTRA CALORIES BURNED
METABOLISM BOOST: ABOUT 10 PERCENT

15 easy ways to up your metabolism

Even before you start exercising, you can use plenty of tricks to eliminate visceral fat, improve your flab-burning metabolic process, and start losing weight fast.

DON'T DIET! The *Men's Health* Diet isn't about eating less, it's about eating more—more nutrition-dense food, to crowd out the empty calories and keep you full all day. That's important, because restricting food will kill your metabolism. It makes your body think, "I'm starving here!" And your body responds by slowing your metabolic rate in order to hold on to existing energy stores. What's worse, if the food shortage (meaning your crash diet) continues, you'll begin burning muscle tissue, which just gives your enemy, visceral fat, a greater advantage. Your metabolism drops even more, and fat goes on to claim even more territory.

> **HOT TIP #71**
>
> **Coffee it up.**
> Athletes who drink caffeine before exercise have 66 percent more glycogen in their muscles, giving them greater endurance.

GO TO BED EARLIER A study in Finland looked at sets of identical twins and discovered that of each set of siblings, the twin who slept less and was under more stress had more visceral fat.

EAT MORE PROTEIN Your body needs protein to maintain lean muscle. In a 2006 study in the *American Journal of Clinical Nutrition*, "The Underappreciated Role of Muscle in Health and Disease," researchers argued that the present recommended daily allowance of protein, 0.36 grams per pound of body weight, was established using obsolete data and is woefully inadequate for an individual doing resistance training. Researchers now recommend an amount between 0.8 and 1 gram per pound of body weight. Add a serving, like 3 ounces of lean meat, 2 tablespoons of nuts, or 8 ounces of low-fat yogurt, to every meal and snack. Plus, research showed that protein can up postmeal calorie burn by as much as 35 percent.

GO ORGANIC WHEN YOU CAN Canadian researchers reported that dieters with the most organochlorines (pollutants from pesticides, which are stored in fat cells) experienced a greater than normal dip in metabolism as they lost weight, perhaps because the toxins interfere with the energy-burning process. In other words, pesticides make it harder to lose pounds. Other research hints that pesticides can trigger weight gain. Of course, it's not always easy to find—or to afford—a whole bunch of organic produce. So you need to know when organic counts, and when it's not that important. Organic onions, avocados, grapefruit? Not necessary. But choose organic when buying celery, peaches, strawberries, apples, blueberries, nectarines, bell peppers, spinach, kale or collard greens, cherries, potatoes, and imported grapes; they tend to have the highest levels of pesticides. A simple rule of thumb: If you can eat the skin, go organic.

> **HOT TIP #72**
>
> **Double your abs.** Canadian researchers determined that your abs work nearly twice as hard when you do a plank with your feet on a Swiss ball instead of on the floor.

GET UP, STAND UP Whether you sit or stand at work may play as big a role in your health and your waistline as your fitness routine. In one study researchers discovered that inactivity (4 hours or more) causes a near shutdown in an enzyme that controls fat and cholesterol metabolism. To keep this enzyme active and increase your fat burning, break up long periods of downtime by standing up—for example, while talking on the phone.

DRINK COLD WATER German researchers found that drinking 6 cups of cold water a day (that's 48 ounces) can raise resting metabolism by about 50 calories daily—enough to shed 5 pounds in a year. The increase may come from the work it takes to heat the water to body temperature. Though the extra calories you burn drinking a single glass don't amount to much, making it a habit can add up to pounds lost with essentially zero additional effort.

EAT THE HEAT It turns out that capsaicin, the compound that gives chili peppers their mouth-searing quality, can also fire up your metabolism. Eating about 1 tablespoon of chopped red or green chilies boosts your body's production of heat and the activity of your sympathetic nervous system (responsible for our fight-or-flight response), according to a study published in the *Journal of Nutritional Science and Vitaminology*. The result: a temporary metabolism spike of about 23 percent. Stock up on chilies to add to meals, and keep a jar of red pepper flakes on hand for topping pizzas, pastas, and stir-fries.

> **HOT TIP #73**
>
> **Sprout a healthy new diet.** Baby broccoli sprouts have 100 times as much cancer-fighting sulforaphane as mature broccoli.

REV UP IN THE MORNING Eating breakfast jump-starts metabolism and keeps energy high all day. It's no accident that those who skip this meal are 4 1/2 times as likely to be obese. And the heartier your first meal is, the better. In one study published by the *American Journal of Epidemiology*, volunteers who got 22 to 55 percent of their total calories at breakfast gained only 1.7 pounds on average over 4 years. Those who ate zero to 11 percent of their calories in the morning gained nearly 3 pounds.

DRINK COFFEE OR TEA Caffeine is a central nervous system stimulant, so your daily java jolt can rev your metabolism 5 to 8 percent—about

98 to 174 calories a day. A cup of brewed tea can raise your metabolism by 12 percent, according to one Japanese study. Researchers believe the antioxidant catechins in tea provide the boost.

FIGHT FAT WITH FIBER Fiber can rev your fat burn by as much as 30 percent. Studies find that those who eat the most fiber gain the least weight over time. Aim for about 25 g a day—the amount in about three servings each of fruits and vegetables.

EAT IRON-RICH FOODS Iron is essential for carrying the oxygen your muscles need to burn fat. Unless you restock your store, you run the risk of low energy and a sagging metabolism. Shellfish, lean meats, beans, fortified cereals, and spinach are excellent sources. (But it's not always a good idea to take a supplement. Too much iron has been linked to a greater risk of heart disease in men. Get this essential mineral in natural doses from real foods.)

GET MORE D Vitamin D is essential for preserving metabolism-revving muscle tissue. Unfortunately, researchers estimate that a measly 20 percent of Americans take in enough through their diet. Get 90 percent of your recommended daily value (400 IU) in a 3.5-ounce serving of salmon. Other good sources: tuna, fortified milk and cereals, and eggs.

DRINK MILK There's some evidence that calcium deficiency may slow metabolism. Research shows that consuming calcium in dairy foods such as fat-free milk and low-fat yogurt may also reduce fat absorption from other foods.

EAT WATERMELON The amino acid arginine, abundant in watermelon, might promote weight loss, according to a new study in the *Journal of Nutrition*. Researchers supplemented the diets of obese mice with arginine over 3 months and found that it decreased body-fat gains by a whopping 64 percent. Adding this amino acid to the diet enhanced the oxidation of fat and glucose and increased lean muscle, which burns more calories than fat does. Snack on watermelon and other arginine sources, such as seafood, nuts, and seeds, year-round.

STAY HYDRATED All of your body's chemical reactions, including your metabolism, depend on water. If you are dehydrated, you may be burning up to 2 percent fewer calories, according to researchers at the University of Utah who monitored the metabolic rates of 10 adults as they drank varying amounts of water per day. In the study, those who drank either eight or twelve 8-ounce glasses of water a day had higher metabolic rates than those who had four.

The long-term calorie burn you get from weight training doesn't just get rid of extra weight. It specifically targets belly fat!

6

THE *MEN'S HEALTH* RULES OF THE RIPPED!
SEVEN SIMPLE RULES THAT WILL SET YOU UP FOR A LIFETIME OF LOOKING GREAT.

Men like rules. Rules are what make things interesting. After all, how much fun would it be if you had endless downs to reach the goal line, if the strike zone were an infinite expanse, or if the only time you got called for a double dribble was when you stopped to gawk at a cheerleader? Not very. Rules are what make the game. Rules are how you know who's winning and who's losing.

That's why I created the *Men's Health* Rules of the Ripped. Once you have a few basic guidelines—incredibly effective, incredibly easy to remember and follow—you can't help but start to see results. And the closer you stick to them, the faster you'll reach your ideal physique.

Seven simple rules. Consider them pledges—pledges to yourself. And you're going to be amazed by just how easy they are to follow. But more amazingly, once you know them, you'll realize that sticking to them every single day isn't even necessary. They're laws, sure, but so is the speed limit. And when's the last time you drove all the way to Grandma's house going 55?

Why the Rules of the Ripped Will Work for You

As I said at the beginning of this book, there's a war going on inside your body, a war between fat and muscle. But in this eternal battle, fat has the advantage. And for that, you can blame Mother Nature.

When humans first evolved, starvation and deprivation were always threats. So our bodies learned to store fat in flush times and burn fewer calories when calories aren't easy to come by—similar to bears preparing for hibernation.

The problem is that today we no longer have to scratch our way across the savannah looking for grubs to eat. Now we're surrounded by grub to eat, stacked on 18-foot-high shelves at the local discount store. And yet, strangely, we still put our bodies in starvation mode more than we might expect. We skip breakfast to race to our jobs. We work long days, breaking to eat only when our bellies rumble. Sometimes, we even go on diets, trying to earn some sort of karmic merit badge by depriving ourselves.

But every time you skip a meal or feel a hunger pang? Your primitive mammalian body feels it, too, and says, "Uh-oh. The big animal isn't getting enough food. Better shuttle some of those Doritos down to the gut region, just in case there's a famine on the horizon."

Literally, every time you let yourself grow hungry, you're telling your body to store fat. That's why each of the Rules of the Ripped is designed to keep you eating—a lot. To melt away fat and build new muscle, you'll need to pack your day with nutrient-rich foods that are both filling and delicious. As you'll discover, all of the guidelines in the *Men's Health* Nutrition System are about eating more food, not depriving yourself of food. Your goal is to pack your body with so much good nutrition that it forgets about the junk calories out there and instead starts to build and maintain new muscle and shed flab.

HOT TIP #74

Rely on Old Yeller. Yellowfin tuna carries mercury levels that are up to 50 percent lower than those of bluefin or bigeye.

Plus, as you follow the Rules of the Ripped, you'll discover that when you eat is almost as important as what you eat. As you begin to work with your body's natural metabolic clock, you'll be shocked to discover how easy it is to lose weight with the *Men's Health* Nutrition System and how fast our plan begins to take effect. In fact, these rules are as flexible as a Vegas showgirl and so simple that even an outlaw can live by them.

RULE 1

"I Will Eat Protein with Every Meal and Every Snack."

Here's why this rule is so important: At any given moment, even at rest, your body is breaking down and building up protein, says Jeff Volek, PhD, RD, a nutrition and exercise researcher at the University of Connecticut. Substitute the word "muscle" for "protein," and you quickly understand just how dynamic your body is and how your muscle content can change considerably in the course of just a few weeks.

But muscle doesn't come just from pumping iron, hauling lumber, or visiting Roger Clemens's "nutritionist." Muscle buildup is triggered by eating protein. In fact, every time you eat at least 10 to 15 grams of protein, you trigger a burst of protein synthesis. And when you eat at least 30 grams, that period of synthesis lasts about 3 hours—and that means even more muscle growth. Here's a quick look at what those numbers translate into when they actually hit your plate.

30 Grams of Protein

1 4-ounce ground beef patty

1 large chicken breast

1 4-ounce sirloin steak

1 large egg vegetable omelet with 3 strips bacon

20 large peel-and-eat wild shrimp

1 lobster

1 haddock fillet

1 6-ounce pork chop

1 6-ounce serving tempeh

10 to 15 Grams of Protein

1 fruit-and-yogurt parfait with granola

2 medium carrots with   cup hummus

cup chili con carne

1 serving spaghetti with meat sauce (10 ounces)

1 pouch chunk light tuna

cup oatmeal with 1 cup 2% milk

12 ounces lowfat chocolate milk

6 ounces Greek yogurt

2 Tbsp peanut butter on whole wheat

Now think about it: When would you typically eat most of your protein? At dinner, right? That means you might be fueling muscle growth for only a few hours a day, mostly while watching *South Park* reruns. The rest of the day, you're breaking down muscle because you don't have enough protein in your system. "The single most important diet upgrade for men who want to lose weight is to eat protein for breakfast," says Louis Aronne, MD, director of the Comprehensive Weight Control Program at New York College Weill Cornell Medical-Presbyterian Hospital. "I've had guys lose a bunch of weight just making this one change."

YOUR PLAN: Eat protein at all three meals, which can include meats and eggs or other options such as cheese and milk. You need to boost your protein intake to between 0.8 and 1.0 gram per pound of body weight in order to preserve your calorie-burning muscle mass. (That's a total of between 148 and 185 grams daily for a 185-pound guy.) That means aiming for approximately 30 grams of protein at your main meals, with filling options like a chicken breast, a hamburger, or a fillet of fish. For each snack, eat at least 10 to 15 grams of protein, such as two hard-boiled eggs, an order of rice and beans, or even a classic peanut butter sandwich on wheat bread. And when in doubt, reach for milk or cheese. Harvard Medical School researchers found that people who ate three servings of dairy daily (1,200 milligrams of calcium) were 60 percent less likely to be overweight than people who consumed less.

HOT TIP #75

Count on Chocula. As few as 30 calories a day of dark chocolate can help lower blood pressure.

TRICK YOURSELF SLIM: Make a snack out of yogurt once a day. Not only does it provide a calcium hit, but a University of Tennessee study also found that people who added three servings of yogurt a day to their diets lost 81 percent more belly fat over 12 weeks than those who didn't eat yogurt. And a study in *Molecular Systems Biology* found that yogurt-based bacteria can prevent the body from absorbing fat. Bugs that eat your fat! Who knew?

RULE 2

"I Will Never Eat the World's Worst Breakfast."

What's the world's worst breakfast?

No breakfast at all.

When you wake up in the morning, your body is fuel deprived. It's been 7 to 9 hours (or more) since you last ate. Your insulin level has dropped, your protein store is empty, and your muscles are as desperate for nutrition as Jimmy Fallon is for laughs. Your body needs food to restore its balance. "The bulk of your calories should come at breakfast," says David Grotto, RD, spokesperson for the American Dietetic Association. "When you shift calories to the morning, you lose weight and keep it off."

It's true. Regularly skipping breakfast increases your risk of obesity by 450 percent. And breakfast is the one meal where, calories be damned, eating more is almost always better than eating less—in an ideal world, you'd get between 500 and 750 calories at breakfast alone. Just make sure some of those calories come from protein. In a 2008 study, researchers at Virginia Commonwealth University found that people who regularly ate a protein-rich, 600-calorie breakfast lost significantly more weight in 8 months than those who consumed only 300 calories and a quarter of the protein. The big breakfast eaters lost an average of 40 pounds and had an easier time sticking with the diet, even though both groups were prescribed about the same number of total daily calories.

> **HOT TIP #76**
>
> **Reach the beach.**
> A stroll on the sand uses more than 2½ times as much energy as regular walking, and builds greater calf strength.

And that's why the world's worst breakfast is no breakfast at all.

Okay, class, I can tell some of you are getting anxious. Heck, you're on the edges of your seats, waving your hands in the air. "Ooh, ooh, I know something worse than nothing for breakfast!" Well, I doubt it. Breakfast is like a paycheck: Lousy is always better than nothing. Go ahead, just try to come up with a breakfast worth skipping...

• *How about...sugar doughnuts!* Okay, not the ideal breakfast solution, but a Sugar-Raised Donut at Dunkin' Donuts is only 230 calories, and with it you're still getting a little protein (3 grams). Add a glass of 2% milk and now you've raised your protein and given yourself a calcium boost, and you're still at just 350 calories. Heck, have another doughnut!

• *How about ... a cup of joe and an Egg McMuffin! Sooo* much better than nothing at all. In fact, the much-maligned McMuffin actually deserves props as one of the few fast-food options with more protein (18 grams) than fat (12 grams). Skip the greasy hash browns and the sugary coffee drinks and get two McMuffins instead. You're still rocking just 600 calories, with a whopping 36 grams of protein.

• *Gotcha now ... a couple slices of cold sausage and pepperoni pizza!* Two leftover slices of Domino's Hand-Tossed sausage and pepperoni—and seriously, if you can choke those down first thing in the morning, you should donate your intestines to science—rack up about 718 calories and 35 grams of fat. But you've got 28 grams of protein from the meat and cheese, calcium from the cheese, carbs for energy from the crust, and even a few vitamins from the tomato sauce. Now consider that in a 2010 study in the *International Journal of Obesity*, adolescents who consumed the most protein at breakfast consumed 130 fewer calories at the subsequent lunch than those who ate the least protein at their morning meal. Makes you wish Papa John's started delivering at 7 a.m., huh?

• *What if ... you took a whole cinnamon bun, fried it, then slathered it in cream cheese, stuffed it with maple syrup ice cream, and doused it in caramel!* Okay, you're really stretching here. What twisted mind could create such a monstrosity? Oh, Friendly's did? And it's on their breakfast menu? And they call it Caramel Cinnamon Swirl French Toast? Damn! Okay, you got me with this one—it's a day's worth of calories (2,090), and a mind-blowing 856 calories of that comes from sugar! Then you've got 57 grams of fat and half a day's sodium intake and relatively little protein. Wow, that really is the world's worst breakfast.

CONCLUSION: If you read and follow the *Men's Health* Nutrition

> **HOT TIP #77**
>
> **Make it sweeter without sweets.** People on low-sugar diets have less depression and anxiety than carb consumers.

System, you'll know exactly how to select a great breakfast that mixes protein, calcium, fiber, carbs, and other nutrients. The better the quality of the food you put in your body, the better the body you'll get in return. But, if it comes down to something sketchy or nothing at all, in most cases, eat what's there and make up for it by eating as healthfully as you can for the rest of the day. And if you are shipwrecked on a deserted island and the only thing left standing from the now-extinct former civilization is an abandoned Friendly's, and the dust-enshrouded freezer unit has just one thing left to eat and it's Caramel Cinnamon Swirl French Toast . . . well, in that case, you're excused from breakfast.

HOT TIP #78

Hangover cure #397. Amino acids in poached eggs help erase next-day hurtin', according to a study in the *Journal of Inflammation Research.*

Otherwise, wake up and start eating!

YOUR PLAN: Eat a considerable portion of your daily calories—30 to 35 percent of your total intake—in the morning. The very best breakfast will match proteins and whole grains with produce and healthy fats. For example: fried eggs on whole-grain toast and a protein-and-fruit smoothie. If you have neither the time nor the stomach for a big breakfast, eat two small ones—have cereal with your coffee, then grab a yogurt and fruit to eat at your desk. But the bottom line is this: Get some protein for breakfast, and the rest of the day will take care of itself.

TRICK YOURSELF SLIM: So you absolutely, positively, no kidding, have zero time for anything but a cup of coffee? Okay: Before you pour the coffee, fill your cup with milk. Drink it down until you have just the right amount to lighten your joe, then add the caffeine. Eight ounces of 1% milk gives you 110 calories and 8 grams of protein, along with a hit of fat-burning calcium. Even if you can't possibly eat breakfast, well, guess what: You just ate breakfast!

RULE 3

"I Will Eat Before and After Exercise."

As in romance, comedy, and the stock market, timing is everything when it comes to food and exercise. And the great news for any guy who loves to eat: You probably need to eat more. In fact, eating more of the right foods at the right times can turn every workout into the best workout of your life.

Indeed, when it comes to exercise and nutrition, researchers are worrying a lot less about the what and thinking a lot more about the when. Here's what eating at the right time can do for you.

• *Build more muscle.* Eating before training speeds muscle growth, according to Dutch and British researchers. In one study, men who ate a protein- and carbohydrate-rich meal right before and right after their workouts built twice as much muscle as men who waited at least 5 hours to eat. By fueling your body with protein and carbohydrates within an hour or two of exercise, you provide your muscles with enough energy to build strength and burn fat more effectively.

• *Burn more fat.* University of Syracuse researchers found that when you down protein before and after weight training, you blunt the effects of cortisol, the stress hormone that tells your body to store fat. As a result, you burn more fat, not only during your workout, but for an additional 24 hours afterward. (Study participants ate a combo of 22 grams of protein and 35 grams of carbs—about what you'd get from a glass of milk and a turkey sandwich.)

> **HOT TIP #79**
>
> **Cow the dentist.**
> Eating yogurt four times a week reduces your risk of cavities by 25 percent.

• *Sculpt your body.* Finnish scientists who had weight lifters drink a protein shake before and after a workout discovered that their subjects produced more of a molecule called cyclin-dependent kinase 2

(CDK2). CDK2 signals your muscles to produce more stem cells, which aid the process of building muscle and improve your body's ability to heal after resistance training. Stem cells are your body's microscopic fountains of youth. The shake drinkers gained more muscle size than their counterparts and had a higher muscle-to-flab ratio than those who didn't take the shakes.

• *Feel more energy—and less pain!* British researchers discovered that a mix of protein and carbs before and after your workout can inhibit muscle breakdown and reduce inflammation. That means you not only build muscle faster, but also recover more quickly and with less next-day soreness.

All this just from eating a little more food? Now that's a diet!

YOUR PLAN: Eat a snack composed of carbohydrates and protein 30 minutes or so before your workout, and eat one of your protein-rich meals immediately after exercise. (One of the mantras we use at *Men's Health* is "Lost time is lost muscle." Your body breaks down muscle during and after exercise to use as fuel and rebuilds muscle using calories that you've consumed. The longer you wait after exercising to eat, the more time your body will spend breaking down its own muscle and the less time you'll have to build new muscle.

TRICK YOURSELF SLIM: A protein shake right after your shower is the fastest nutrition delivery system there is. You can even download our Smoothie Selector app at menshealth.com/apps.

HOT TIP #80

Get clean, get lean. You don't need liposuction to vacuum off the fat. In an Indiana University study, people with the cleanest houses had the highest levels of physical activity. "It could be that these people burn a lot of extra calories keeping their homes clean," says study author NiCole Keith, PhD.

RULE 4

"I Will Eat It If It Grows on a Tree."

Or a bush, stalk, or vine, as well. In other words, if it grows on or is a plant, eat it. Fruits and vegetables should be included in every meal and as many snacks as possible. The reason: Your goal is to fill your body with muscle-promoting, fat-discouraging nutrients, and the very best source of them is fruits, nuts, and vegetables. By loading your body with the maximum amount of nutrients for the least number of calories, they're a dietary bargain. A study at UCLA found that the typical person of normal weight consumed two servings of fruit a day, on average, while the typical overweight person ate just one piece. Another study in the journal *Appetite* found that eating whole fruit at the beginning of a meal reduces your overall calorie intake by 15 percent. Now, a caveat here: Eating "vegetable chips" or "veggie sticks" or drinking "fruit-flavored punch" is not the same thing. If the fruit or vegetable in question won't wilt or rot after a few days of hanging out on your countertop, then it's a processed food. It didn't grow from the ground, it grew out of some scientist's imagination.

Another benefit to eating off the trees: You'll get more heart-healthy omega-3 fatty acids. Some experts argue that omega-3s should be labeled an essential nutrient, as necessary to health as, say, vitamins A and D. "They're involved in the metabolism of each individual cell," says Artemis P. Simopoulos, MD, president of the Center for Genetics, Nutrition and Health in Washington, DC. "They're part of your body's basic nutrition." Studies show that this healthy fat may not only reduce a person's risk of heart disease and stroke, but also possibly help prevent ailments as diverse as arthritis, Alzheimer's disease, asthma, autoimmune disorders, and attention-deficit/hyperactivity disorder—and those are just the As. On top of its mood-boosting, heart-saving, brain-enhancing powers, those who consume the most omega-3-rich foods live longer and carry less abdominal fat than those who eat the least. And scientists from Quebec found that omega-3s improve protein metabolism, meaning that more of the protein you eat is synthesized in your muscle tissue. Sure it sounds cool, but even better, this means faster muscle growth.

> **HOT TIP #81**
>
> **Envision success.** University of Iowa scientists found that people who monitored their diet and exercise goals most frequently were more likely to achieve them than people who set goals but rarely reviewed them.

You already know that you can find this healthy fat in fatty fish like salmon and tuna, but it's also found growing in trees: Two highly potent sources of omega-3s are walnuts and kiwifruit. (Keep a container of ground flaxseed in your kitchen as well; it's extremely high in omega-3s and adds a nutty flavor to smoothies, PB&J sandwiches, and salads.)

YOUR PLAN: Eat at least one serving of fruits or vegetables at every meal. You can and should eat as much of them as you want to help satisfy cravings.

TRICK YOURSELF SLIM: Eat your fruits and vegetables first! Not only will you consume more vegetables and fewer calories from other foods, but the fiber content will lower the glycemic load of your meal, helping you sidestep those swings in blood sugar that lead to hunger. Try at least one new fruit or vegetable each week, and make sure that salads and fruit salads have at least four different colors. For example: lettuce, yellow peppers, tomatoes, and carrots; or pineapple, blood oranges, kiwi, and grapes.

RULE 5

"I Will Eat the Salad Even If It Makes Me Feel Girly."

What could be more manly than green, leafy foliage—the stuff of the woods, the jungle, the open range, the outfield at Wrigley Field? Who came up with the idea that salads were wimpy?

For generations, hunters and soldiers have covered the outsides of their bodies in leafy greens, all the better to stalk their prey. Yet for some reason, we see a leaf on a dinner plate and we're offended, as if eating it were somehow an affront to our manhood. Does that make any sense?

The confusion started when some crazy-eyed dietitian tried to convince us to eat salads instead of real food like burgers and ribs. Bad dietitian! A man should eat salads not in place of his other foods, but rather in addition to them. (That's right, continue eating, but now eat more.) The reason is that salads deliver wildly important nutrients that are hard to come by elsewhere—nutrients that help promote weight loss.

EXAMPLE: Folate, a B vitamin found primarily in leafy greens, is perhaps the best indicator of how healthy your diet really is. Folate deficiency is linked to most of the major diseases of our time: It leads to increased risks of stroke, heart disease, obesity, cognitive impairment, Alzheimer's disease, cancer, and depression as well as a decreased response to depression treatments. (Folate is the anti-fat-and-stupid vitamin.) Some of the best food sources of

> **HOT TIP #82**
>
> **Sip up, sit up.**
> You can do 17 percent more reps when you're well-hydrated, say researchers at the University of Connecticut.

folate are foods you're not going to eat a lot of, no matter how often you're told to—kale, Swiss chard, and collard greens. Had any lately? No? Then it's that much more important that you order the salad, leaning whenever possible toward romaine or spinach. It's hard to get enough folate. Other sources are broccoli, brussels sprouts, lentils, beans, liver, and peas—again, not exactly a roll call of man's favorite foods. But they're worth it: A study in the *British Journal of Nutrition* found that dieters who ate the most folate were able to lose 8½ times as much weight as those who ate the least.

YOUR PLAN: At every meal, try to include a folate-rich food. The best way to up your folate intake is to eat leafy greens with as many meals as you can, and eat them first.

TRICK YOURSELF SLIM: Make a salad dressing with mustard, vinegar, and safflower oil. In a study in the *American Journal of Clinical Nutrition*, researchers found that the high amount of linoleic acid in safflower oil may keep your body from storing fat.

RULE 6

"I Will Not Drink Sugar Water."

This ought to be the easiest rule to stick to, right? After all, when was the last time you drank sugar water?

If you're like most American men, the answer is: earlier today. In fact, the average guy in the United States consumes more than 7 percent of his daily calories from sugar water—about a gallon of the stuff, and hundreds of calories, every day. How is that possible? Well, sugar water makes up the majority of the soft drinks we consume each day. Here are some common sugar waters that you might have enjoyed recently.

COLA: sugar water + caramel coloring and flavoring
A typical cola is about 89 percent carbonated water and 9 percent high fructose corn syrup (HFCS).

SWEETENED ICED TEA: sugar water + tea
Teas like Snapple are about 89 percent water and 10 percent HFCS.

VITAMIN WATER: sugar water + chemical forms of vitamins

One of the worst things to happen to both water and vitamins. An average brand is 92 percent water and more than 5 percent sugar.

FRUIT DRINKS: sugar water + fruit juice

If your juice has the word "cocktail" attached to it, it's about 63 percent water, 27 percent juice, and more than 9 percent HFCS.

ENERGY DRINKS: sugar water + caffeine and herbs

They list plenty of mysterious ingredients like taurine and guarana and milk thistle, but the average energy drink is 84.5 percent water and 12.3 percent sugar.

In fact, the average American now drinks more than 450 calories every day. By cutting that amount in half you would cut enough calories to lose about 25 pounds in a year. Plus, you'd be cutting down on fructose, a type of sugar that's coming under more scrutiny every year. In 2010, Robert Lustig, MD, professor of clinical pediatrics at the University of California–San Francisco, discovered that fructose has much the same effect on the human body as alcohol, including causing the same kind of liver scarring that is found in alcoholics. (Table sugar and high-fructose corn syrup are both about 50 percent fructose.)

> **HOT TIP #83**
>
> **Root for the reds.**
> Red cabbage has 15 times as much wrinkle-fighting beta-carotene as green cabbage. Red bell peppers have nine times as much as the green ones.

YOUR PLAN: Replace sodas, iced teas, and "performance beverages" with water, seltzer, or other low-calorie or calorie-free beverages. (And don't just change over to the "diet" version of your favorite soft drink. You'll read why below.) If you don't like the taste of your water, buy a home filter (like Brita), which will help take out any chemical tastes, and keep a container of it cold in your fridge. Researchers from the University of Utah found that the people who drink the most water have the highest metabolisms. In a study, subjects drank 4, 8, or 12 cups of water each day. Those who drank at least 8 cups reported better concentration and higher energy levels, and tests showed that they were burning calories at much higher rates than the 4-cups-a-day group.

TRICK YOURSELF SLIM: Drink the moment you wake up. The legendary Gracie family—the family that invented Brazilian jiu-jitsu—lives by a code of always being ready to fight. And the first thing every Gracie does when he or she wakes up is drink a big glass of water, because being ready to fight means being properly hydrated. Now it turns out that their tradition makes sense even for those of us who don't like getting punched in the face repeatedly. A study in the *Journal of the American Dietetic Association* found that drinking a glass of water before breakfast can cut daily food intake by 13 percent. So on top of the calories you're saving by swapping soda for H$_2$O, you're saving another 200 or so by staving off hunger pangs! (That's another 21 pounds gone in a year!)

HOT TIP #84

Make a pit stop.
Natural anti-inflammatories in olives suppress the same pain pathways as over-the counter ibuprofen.

A CAVEAT: You'd think the easiest way to cut out sugar water calories would be to switch to diet sodas and teas. And yes, that will cut calories. But for reasons we don't fully grasp, diet sodas actually increase your risk of weight gain. Research shows that people who drink one to two cans of regular soda per day increase their risk of becoming overweight or obese by nearly 33 percent. But replace those regular sodas with diet sodas and the risk rises: diet drinkers are 65 percent are more likely to become overweight, and 41 percent more likely to become obese. Several studies have hinted at why this is. In 2009, researchers found that artificial sweeteners may interfere with your brain's satisfaction signals, essentially making you crave more food than you need. And even more recent research by scientists in the Department of Psychological Sciences at Purdue University suggests that artificial sweeteners may slow metabolism—meaning the more diet soda you drink, the fewer calories you burn during the day.

RULE 7

"I Will Follow the Rules of the Ripped ~~100 Percent~~ 80 Percent of the Time."

If you make the right food choices 80 percent of the time, you can't help but stay lean. That means that one out of every five times you step up to the nutritional tee, you get to shank one—into the ham and cheese sand trap, into Black Forest cake woods. It happens, because nobody's perfect—and not trying to be perfect is one of the keys to long-term success. Guys who try to be perfect eventually go crazy, and the next thing you know they're driving their SUVs into fire hydrants while being chased by angry blondes wielding 9-irons.

Don't try to be perfect. Be 80 percent. That'll still put you ahead of most of the adult male population. And more important, it will send you on your way to the body you've always wanted. In Chapter 10, you'll find a list of the 250 Best Foods for Men. If you want a chocolate bar make sure it's the best one. (Dagoba's Beaucoup Berries bar, which mixes in cherries and cranberries to pack in a whopping 7 grams of fiber for just 250 calories.) Craving a steak? Go get one, but make the very best choice. (At Ruby Tuesday, you can order a plain grilled top sirloin with just 391 calories—ordering it "plain" will strip off 1,000 milligrams of sodium.) Make a peanut butter and jelly sandwich,

> **HOT TIP #85**
>
> **Beware your buddies.** Men eat 35 percent more calories when they're with male friends than with female companions.

but use the best PB, the best J, and the best bread in the world.

You'll be stunned by how effective this strategy is. Let's look at a potential 3-day menu. Say, for instance, that Friday night you went out and ate a burger from a chain restaurant; on Saturday night, you went out and got ribs; and on Sunday night, you heated up a frozen pizza while watching the game. On each of the 3 mornings you had a bowl of cereal, and lunch was a modest cup of yogurt and a piece of fruit. Here's what the difference might be if you ate the very best foods, instead of the worst.

BEST	WORST	SAVINGS
BURGER McDonald's Big N' Tasty (hold the mayo) 410 calories	Cheesecake Factory Ranch House Burger 1,941 calories	**1,531 calories**
RIBS (½ rack) Ruby Tuesday's Memphis Dry Rub Baby-Back 460 calories	Applebee's Double-Glazed Baby Back Ribs 1000 calories	**540 calories**
FROZEN PIZZA (⅓ pie) Amy's Cheese Pizza 290 calories	Digiorno for Lunch Traditional Crust Supreme Pizza 790 calories	**500 calories**
CEREAL Kashi Whole Wheat Biscuits, Cinnamon Harvest 180 calories	Quaker Natural Granola with Raisins (1 cup) 420 calories	**240 calories (x3!)**
YOGURT Stonyfield Oikos Plain Greek Yogurt 80 calories	Yoplait Original 99% Fat Free Strawberry 170 calories	**90 calories (x3!)**
Total calories saved in just one weekend:		**3,561!**

NOW CONSIDER THIS: It takes 3,500 calories to build a pound of fat. In the course of just 72 hours, by eating the exact same foods, just better versions of them, you've actually saved more than a pound of fat! Do that every weekend for a year—and remember, you're still eating ribs, burgers, and pizza—and you've shed 52 pounds of flab. (And that's without even changing how you eat on weekdays!)

Amazing, right? Do your best to follow the *Men's Health* Nutrition System 80 percent of the time, shoot for the 250 Best Foods for Men whenever you need a break, and you've got this fat thing solved. More than 80 percent? You'll be downright Schwarzeneggerian!

TRICK YOURSELF SLIM: If you want to eat something that's really, truly horrible for you (like, you can't stop thinking about the Friendly's Caramel Cinnamon Swirl French Toast mentioned earlier), wash it down with a glass of milk. A study in the *American Journal of Clinical Nutrition* found that those who consume calcium from dairy every day decrease the levels of triacylglycerol in their blood (a major form of fat in the circulatory system) by 15 to 19 percent.

A WORD ABOUT COUNTING CALORIES

No matter how healthy you eat, consuming more calories than your body burns is a surefire route to weight gain. That's why many diet plans are based on counting calories, using very tightly managed caloric calculations to ensure that dieters never go over their allotted food intake.

At *Men's Health,* we've spent the last 2 decades studying calorie-counting systems, using the absolute best science, soliciting the finest mathematical minds, and boiling these intensely intricate scientific findings into an equation any guy can understand. The ultimate calorie-intake formula for men looks like this:

$$\text{Caloric intake} \times \text{BMI}^2 \div \text{waist circumference} - (3{,}500 \div (24 + 7)) = \$*\&\%\# \text{ BORING!}$$

Look, we're guys. We figure out how much to eat the same way we figure out whether we need an iron or a wood, whether we're swinging at a fastball or a changeup, and whether she's a 7 or a 10: We eyeball it. Sometimes we hit it a little too hard, sometimes not hard enough, but we trust that, over time, it'll even out.

But over the past 30 years, food marketers have tricked out their offerings, throwing us sidearm curves and knuckleballs and other pitches that don't look at all like they're supposed to. The problem is most egregious at America's restaurants, where they now market meal-size plates as appetizers, family-size platters as single entrées, and small kiddie pools as beverages. A 2008 study by the USDA found that Americans eat an average of 107 more calories each time they choose to eat at a restaurant instead of at home. And a 2002 study looking at restaurant portions found that the average restaurant pasta dish was nearly five times bigger than the USDA's recommended serving! Steaks and bagels were more than three times as big as one serving should be, and hamburgers more than double.

So how can the average guy defend himself against calorie counts and serving sizes that are ballooning faster than the national debt? How can you become a nutritional cost cutter, paring back excess caloric spending while still getting the fat, protein, fiber, and other nutrients you need? And how can you do it all the same way you pick out a golf club—by eyeballing it?

The answer is in the palm of your hand. Literally.

For solid foods, a serving size is equal to:

MEATS: The size of your palm

VEGETABLES AND FRUITS: As big as a tight fist

OILS AND OTHER HEALTHY FATS: A teaspoon is the end of your thumb, from the knuckle up

LEGUMES: Whatever fits in the palm of your hand

GRAINS: The size of a tight fist

DAIRY: The size of your palm

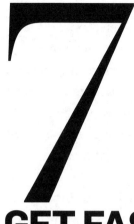

GET FAST & LEAN!
DISCOVER THE EIGHT SUPERFOOD GROUPS IN THE *MEN'S HEALTH* NUTRITION SYSTEM THAT WILL TURBO-CHARGE YOUR WEIGHT-LOSS PLANS!

As any guy who's ever reenacted the cafeteria scene in *Animal House* knows, food can make for a powerful weapon. A cold, greasy fry applied smartly to the cheek or an over-ripe tomato delivered to the back of the head can have a serious impact on one's chosen adversary. But chances are that it's been a long time since you last launched a food grenade at an unsuspecting diner. (And if not, then you probably don't get invited to a lot of dinner parties anymore.)

Well, it's time to channel your inner Blutarsky and declare a food fight once again. But this time, you're not battling the pointy-headed Neidermeyers of the world; this time, you're going to be waging a food fight against an even more insidious enemy: belly fat. This chapter will introduce you to your weapons of choice.

Several years ago, *Men's Health* Editor-in-Chief David Zinczenko wrote the groundbreaking book *The Abs Diet*, in which he listed a dozen critical food groups that play a role in boosting metabolism. The *Men's Health* Nutrition System simplifies that concept. By focusing on just these eight types of foods, you'll be eating—and looking—fast and lean, which is why we grouped them in just this way. FAST & LEAN is the simple acronym to remember: Everything you'll find on this list is choice body-chiseling chow. Anything you eat that doesn't fall into one of these categories, on the other hand, probably isn't good for you. To maximize muscle growth and fat burn, just hit the suggested serving scores. You'll fuel your body with all the nutrients it needs, and you'll crowd out the bad foods in the process.

THE SUPERFOOD DAILY BOX SCORE

FIBER-RICH GRAINS − 1 servings
AVOCADOS, OILS, AND OTHER HEALTHY FATS = 1 to 2 servings
SPINACH AND OTHER LEAFY GREENS = 4 or more servings
TURKEY AND OTHER LEAN MEATS = 2 servings
&
LEGUMES = 1 or more serving
EGGS AND DAIRY = 3 to 5 servings
APPLES AND OTHER FRUITS = 3 or more servings
NUTS AND SEEDS = 1 or more serving

The *Men's Health* FAST & LEAN Superfoods

These eight food groups have been specifically selected for their fat-fighting properties. Here's some of the science behind the magic.

Fiber-rich grains

THE HIGHLIGHTS: Has years of bad nutritional information caused you to react to carbs the way citizens of Tokyo react to Godzilla? Calm down! There's nothing inherently wrong with carbohydrates, until food scientists get hold of them and turn them bright orange, electric lavender, or fluorescent green. Healthy carbs like whole grains, pasta, and pitas can and should be staples of your daily diet. They provide energy, help facilitate the muscle-building process, and reduce your risk of one of man's biggest enemies: prostate cancer. Whole-grain breads and pastas and brown rice are obvious choices. But stretch out: Quinoa and oats are packed with fiber and are so protein-rich they practically count as meat!

THE SCIENCEY STUFF: Researchers at Pennsylvania State University compared those who ate whole grains to those who ate refined grains, and found that whole-grain eaters lost 2.4 times more belly fat than those who ate refined grains. The high fiber helps, but these results go beyond simple satiety. Whole grains more favorably affect blood glucose levels, which means there aren't wild swings in your blood sugar that ratchet up cravings after you eat them. Plus, the antioxidants in whole grains help control inflammation and insulin (the hormone that tells your body to store fat).

YOUR GOAL: Four servings of whole grains per day, aiming to eat at least one serving both before and after your workout.

CAVEAT: When it comes to carbs, food manufacturers love to mess with our heads. They refine our wheat, rice, and other grains, stripping out all the vitamins, minerals, and fiber found in the bran (the outside of the grain) and the germ (the very center), and leaving the nutritionally dead endosperm—which they then spray with chemical facsimiles of nutrients and call "enriched." (To get an idea of what this looks like, think of a kernel of corn. The skin on the outside is the bran, and the little tiny seed in the middle is the germ. Everything else is the endosperm.) So when you see "multigrain" or "wheat" on the label of a loaf of bread or cereal, you probably think, "Ah, the healthy stuff!" But read the nutrition label. Often, "multigrain" just means more than one grain has had the nutritional life beaten out of it. "Wheat" bread, on the other hand, is often refined white bread that's been dyed with molasses to look healthier for you. Always read the label and always look for "whole grain." If you see the word "refined," don't be refined at all—toss it and run.

Avocados, oils, and other healthy fats

THE HIGHLIGHTS: Here's a nutritional mantra worth remembering: Eating fat won't make you fat any more than eating money will make you rich. Indeed, the right kinds of fats can actually make you slimmer. Your body is designed to burn fat for energy. So by timing your fat intake, you'll not only trigger weight loss, but also fuel your workouts more effectively—and see even greater gains in the gym.

THE SCIENCEY STUFF: The fats we want you to concentrate on are: monounsaturated fats, the healthy oils found in olives, nuts, seeds, avocados, acai fruit, and even chocolate; and omega-3 fatty acids, which are found in cold water fish, grass-fed meats, nuts, seeds, and some fruits. These fats can lower your risk of heart disease, protect cells from damage, help encourage muscle growth, and increase the amounts of valuable nutrients available from other foods. But more shockingly, scientists in Italy found that men who eat diets with higher amounts of fat burn more blubber during exercise. And, in a study in the *International Journal of Obesity*, researchers at Brigham and Women's Hospital in Boston put 101 overweight people on either a low-fat diet or a moderate-fat diet, and followed them for 18 months. Both groups lost weight, but only the moderate-fat group lost an average of 9 pounds per person and kept it off after a year. The reason: Fat consumption helps boost levels of a hormone called leptin, the "satiation hormone" that tells you when you're full.

YOUR GOAL: One to two servings per day. That might include some guacamole, some pasta with olive oil, some salad dressing. Note: You'll also be getting healthy monounsaturated fats from nuts (you'll read more about them in a moment). While you want to eat plenty of those, make sure you're also getting enough healthy fats from the above sources as well.

> **HOT TIP #86**
>
> **De-stress with sex.** In a study of people engaged in public speaking, those who had intercourse in the weeks prior had less severe spikes in blood pressure. Flying solo gave only half the benefits.

Spinach and other leafy greens

THE HIGHLIGHTS: If there's one food group on the *Men's Health* FAST & LEAN list that has almost unlimited benefits, it's leafy green vegetables. Packed with supernutrients that can improve heart health, elevate your mood, burn off calories, and do everything from protect your eyes to boost your sexual potency, vegetables are the best nutritional bargain in the universe. Eat them wherever and whenever you see them.

THE SCIENCEY STUFF: The caloric value of most vegetables is so low that the simple process of eating and digesting greens burns almost as many calories as are in the food. Need more proof? Researchers in New York surveyed more than 2,000 dieters, and those who were most successful, felt the fullest, and lost the most weight ate at least four servings of vegetables per day. Plus, vegetables—especially green, leafy ones like spinach and brussels sprouts—are packed with folate. As you read in the previous chapter, folate, a B vitamin, is the holy grail of nutrients. Scientists believe that the best way to tell if you're eating a healthy diet is to measure your level of this nutrient. Folate is getting harder and harder for Americans to come by as we move away from vegetables and toward more packaged and processed foods. But folate has been shown to fight depression and weight gain. Indeed, in one study, dieters with the highest levels of folate lost 8½ times as much weight as those with the lowest levels.

HOT TIP #87

Go yellow. Yellow split peas are not only higher in protein (16 grams per cup) than green split peas, but studies show that protein might reduce blood pressure. So make a big pot of yellow pea soup.

YOUR GOAL: At least four servings of vegetables each day, including fresh and frozen varieties. (But I'd prefer you eat more—vegetables are like a "get out of the hospital free" card. Don't like vegetables? What are you, 3? Suck it up!) The easiest way to hit this number? Have a salad before your meal whenever you can.

Turkey and other lean meats

THE HIGHLIGHTS: Protein is the basic building block of the entire human body, and meats and eggs are the best sources of it. While eating more protein is a key component of building muscle, it's also your best friend in terms of dramatic body transformation and overall health. Protein does everything from stretching your shirtsleeves to cutting inches from your waist. That's because your body burns a lot of calories when it's digesting protein—about 25 calories for every 100 calories you eat (compared with only 10 to 15 calories for fats and carbs). That's called the thermic effect of eating, and it's where up to 30 percent of our calories get used up. So the more you eat, the more you burn!

THE SCIENCEY STUFF: Protein is made of amino acids, which can be split into two types: essential and nonessential. The best forms of protein include all nine essential amino acids that your body can't naturally produce. Based on this, the ideal protein sources include beef, pork, poultry, fish, dairy, eggs, nuts, and oats. Other sources such as beans, seeds, and cornmeal provide a shot of protein, but the amounts of essential amino acids in these foods fall slightly below your body's needs. Foods like breads, rice, pasta, and potatoes contain protein, but they don't contain the essential amino acids and thus are incomplete sources. A diet that primarily consists of proteins from complete sources will provide the best results.

YOUR GOAL: Two servings per day, focusing especially on breakfast. Be sure to eat something from this category (or from the protein-rich dairy or egg categories) as part of your preworkout and postworkout meals.

Legumes

THE HIGHLIGHTS: What, exactly, is a legume? It's anything that grows inside of a pod, like beans, lentils, peas, edamame, peanuts, and those clones from *Invasion of the Body Snatchers*. With the exception of that last entry, legumes are basically little weight-loss pills. Every time you pop one, you're getting closer to your goal. Try to think of them that way, and you'll find yourself noshing pea soup, grabbing some bean dip, buying bean burritos, and spreading peanut butter on everything.

THE SCIENCEY STUFF: One study found that people who ate ¾ cup of beans daily weighed 6.6 pounds less than those who didn't eat beans, even though the bean eaters consumed 199 more calories per day. (See? Eat more, weigh less.) Another study in the *Journal* *of the American College of Nutrition* discovered that people who eat beans each day have smaller waists and lower blood pressure. And while high doses of soy aren't a good idea, especially for men—soy contains naturally occurring chemicals that mimic estrogen and lower testosterone—the things to avoid are soy oils and additives. Edamame, with its fiber and protein, is still a smart snack choice.

YOUR GOAL: Look to eat at least one serving a day from this category. But remember: They are weight-loss pills, with absolutely no nutritional downside. The more you can eat, the more fat you will lose and the more muscle you will build.

Eggs and dairy

THE HIGHLIGHTS: Turns out that milk does a body good—and so do cheese, yogurt, and even ice cream. Most people know that the calcium in dairy strengthens your bones, but the list of benefits is longer than the wine menu at a snooty French restaurant. Something as simple as drinking a glass of milk per day can help stave off heart attack and stroke. When British researchers looked at the dietary habits of men, those who drank milk at least once per day had a 16 percent lower risk of heart disease and were 20 percent less likely to have a stroke. The calcium in dairy lowers your blood pressure and creates a healthier environment for your heart. Another study, at Harvard Medical School, found that people who ate three servings of dairy foods daily were 60 percent less likely to be overweight than people who consumed less.

Eggs, meanwhile, are the most nutrient-dense food known to man. A study published in the *International Journal of Obesity* found that, compared to those who ate a bagel, dieters who ate a breakfast of eggs (yolk and all) for 5 weeks lost 65 percent more weight—with no effect on their cholesterol or triglycerides. (That's right, eggs are high in cholesterol, but they won't raise your cholesterol—that's a common misconception.)

THE SCIENCEY STUFF: A study at the University of Minnesota found that half of all men don't consume enough vitamin D in their diets, a nutrient that's added to most dairy products. Vitamin D is important because a deficiency can make it harder for you to lose weight. So drink your milk, but don't be afraid to reach for the whole milk. The smoother, tastier version not only suppresses your appetite, but also is healthy. A major review published in the *American Journal of Clinical Nutrition* found no association between the saturated fat in whole milk and clogged coronary arteries. And there's no need to sweat the calories: The difference between whole and 1% or 2% milk is a paltry 20 calories. In addition, researchers in Sweden found that conjugated linoleic acids (CLA), which are found in dairy and beef fat, can decrease waist size. The study followed 25 men—some of them taking a CLA supplement—for 4 weeks, and at the end, the CLA group had

> **HOT TIP #88**
>
> **Go low fat for love.** Switching from super-fatty to lean meats can lift your libido and increase your stamina in the sack.

significantly smaller bellies. (Treat yourself right: Get grass-fed beef and milk whenever possible. Grass-fed beef contains 60 percent more omega-3s, 200 percent more vitamin E, and two to three times as much CLA.)

And while you're seeking out more dairy, focus on yogurt. A University of Tennessee study found that people who added three servings of yogurt a day to their diets lost 81 percent more belly fat over 12 weeks than those who didn't eat yogurt. While calcium played a role, a study in *Molecular Systems Biology* found that yogurt-based bacteria can actually prevent the body from absorbing fat. Try Horizon brand—it contains the same bacterium used in the study.

YOUR GOAL: Three to five servings per day. Be sure to eat something from this category (or from the protein-rich lean meats, legumes, and nuts categories) as part of your preworkout and postworkout meals. Eat eggs for breakfast regularly; munch on cheese at lunchtime; squeeze a yogurt in as a snack whenever you can.

THE BIG QUESTION: Whole, 1% or 2%, or fat-free? In most cases, there's no reason not to go with whole fat. Plenty of evidence shows that fat helps quench your appetite and results in your eating fewer calories during the rest of the day. But fat does something else in dairy products: It prevents the need for added sugars. For example, here's the breakdown for 8 ounces of three types of plain yogurt, from the USDA National Nutrient Database.

	PLAIN, WHOLE MILK	PLAIN, LOW FAT	PLAIN, FAT FREE
SUGARS	10.58 grams	17.25 grams	17.43 grams
CALORIES	138	143	127

By far, the smartest choice here is whole-milk yogurt. It has 39 percent less sugar and a mere 11 calories more than fat-free yogurt, and it actually has fewer calories than low-fat yogurt. And this is only comparing the most innocent of yogurts, the plain variety. Once you start to add fruit flavorings, many low-fat and fat-free yogurts approach 30 grams of sugar per 8-ounce serving. Yoplait Original 99% Fat Free Strawberry, for example, delivers 27 grams of sugar per 6-ounce serving—more than a Kit Kat bar!

Apples and other fruits

THE HIGHLIGHTS: As a good rule of thumb, the more colorful your diet, the healthier you're probably eating. That's because color = nutrition. And the easiest (and tastiest) way to get color into your diet is to eat a variety of fruits—red apples, yellow pineapples, green kiwis, orange, um, oranges. Different colors represent different nutrients, so the wider the variety, the better.

THE SCIENCEY STUFF: Fruits contain natural sugars that, when broken down by your body, are synthesized in your liver. This may sound like technical nonsense, but it's an important benefit for your waistline. Because the sugar is processed in your liver, it doesn't spike your insulin levels, meaning you're less likely to store this energy as fat. Select any of your favorite fruits—either fresh or frozen—and use them as daily snacks or as energy boosters before or after your workouts.

YOUR GOAL: Three or more servings of fruit each day, including fresh, frozen, and dried fruits. This is not hard. Have some raisin bran, eat an apple, and grab a couple of pineapple chunks off the salad bar. You're done.

Nuts and seeds

THE HIGHLIGHTS: Hunger-quenching fiber. Muscle-building protein. Disease-fighting vitamins. Heart-healthy, stomach-satisfying monounsaturated fats. As in *One Flew Over the Cuckoo's Nest,* when it comes to nutrition, the nuts are the sanest guys in the room. Which should you eat? Mix and match them: Walnuts are higher in omega-3 fatty acids than even salmon; hazelnuts boast the muscle-building amino acid arginine; pecans have the highest antioxidant count of any nut; almonds are nature's version of vitamin E supplements. Seeds like those of pumpkins and sunflowers are packed with E and healthy fats as well.

> **HOT TIP #89**
>
> **Feed your hunger, look younger.**
> People who reported having sex four times a week looked 10 years younger than they actually are, according to a 10-year study of 3,500 adults.

THE SCIENCEY STUFF: When researchers at Purdue University had people eat 2 ounces of almonds (about 48) a day for 23 weeks, they found that they not only did not gain weight, but also decreased their caloric intake from unhealthy food sources while improving cardiovascular risk factors like lipid metabolism and cholesterol levels. And researchers from Georgia Southern University found that eating a high-protein, high-fat snack such as almonds increases your resting calorie burn for up to 3½ hours. Another study found that people who ate pistachios for 3 months lost an average of 10 to 12 pounds. According to a study in the *Journal of Nutrition*, you can snack on nuts without worrying about accumulating extra pounds because the body doesn't absorb all the fat in nuts.

YOUR GOAL: Shoot for at least one serving a day from this category.

The *Men's Health* Nutrition System in Action

Here's a quick look at your daily diet plan. (Yep, it's a lot of food!)

BREAKFAST(S)

FOCUS ON: Dairy, eggs, whole grains, fiber, and eating a lot of calories

When you shift calorie intake to the morning, you lose weight and keep it off. So eat a large portion of your daily calories—30 to 35 percent of your total intake—in the early part of the day. If you usually skip breakfast, ease into it with something very light, like a slice of cheese or a glass of milk with whole-wheat toast. Just make sure you start your day with some protein and some carbohydrates. The protein and carbs in dairy slow muscle protein breakdown, promoting muscle growth and fat loss, lessening muscle damage, and reducing inflammation. And, according to Australian scientists, drinking milk for breakfast limits afternoon and nighttime binges. You'll discover that you'll actually eat fewer calories throughout the day if you eat more of them in the morning, and you'll lose more weight simply by eating two breakfasts every day. That's right—you'll lose weight if you eat more.

So, why the "(s)" in "Breakfast(s)"? Because if you don't have the time or appetite to eat a big meal first thing in the morning, you still want to shift as many of your calories to the first third of the day as possible. So if all you can manage is a glass of milk when you first get up, give your brain and your body a boost an hour later by eating a protein-packed meal that includes vegetables or fruits for mood-boosting brainpower. Have walnut flaxseed oatmeal with some yogurt and blueberries for a shot of omega-3s and brain-boosting antioxidants. If you're about to hit the gym, a protein-packed smoothie combining fruits and a scoop of whey powder might be your best bet.

LUNCH

FOCUS ON: Vegetables, beans, fruits, nuts, whole grains, and packing in as much nutrition as possible

Lunch is the defining moment of your nutritional day. Breakfast is all about eating as much as you can; by dinner, the day's shot. It's at lunchtime where everything comes together. It's also the meal where we have the least control over our food intake, especially at work. So be smart: Aim for a lunch that has at least three representatives from the fruits, vegetables, or legumes category—they're mainly water, fiber, and vitamins, so they will keep you hydrated and full with healthy calories. Salads and soups are the easy choices here. Then add in some combination of high-quality proteins, healthy fats, dairy, nuts, and whole grains.

DINNER

FOCUS ON: Leafy greens and other vegetables, lean meats, fish, beans, and legumes; focus also on keeping portion sizes down

Studies show that if you start your dinner with a small side salad dressed with olive oil and vinegar or with steamed folate-rich vegetables like kale, spinach, collard greens, or Swiss chard, you'll decrease your overall food intake by 12 percent while taking in satiating fiber and disease-fighting nutrients. Plus, folate-rich greens will give you a mood boost. Got that? Either eat a salad before dinner or put vegetables on your plate and eat those first. Then you can move on to the main course of lean meats, whole grains, and the like. Twice a week, eat fish, which is rich in omega-3s. Fish will lower your risk of heart disease, protect your cells from damage, and increase the amounts of valuable nutrients your body can absorb from other foods.

SNACKS

FOCUS ON: Dairy, protein, whole grains, fruits, nuts, beans, and legumes

You can't lose weight and keep it off unless you snack! In fact, studies show that people who avoid eating between meals may end up consuming more calories overall, mostly because hungry people make bad food choices. Think protein, think fat, think calcium—your snacks are where you should try to squeeze in extra servings of dairy. Choose plain yogurt and blueberries, red bell pepper slices and cottage cheese, whole-grain cereal and milk, apples and cheese, guacamole and tortilla chips, and walnuts and raspberries.

PRE- AND POST WORKOUT FOODS

FOCUS ON: Dairy, lean meats, whole grains, and nuts (eat before and immediately after exercise)

Do you have to work out? No.

Then again, do you have to save for retirement? Do you have to check the tires on your car for safety? Do you have to spend time with your kids? No. You don't have to do anything if you don't want to. Go lay down on the couch, order a pizza, and keep up with the Kardashians if you want.

But you're a grown man. You understand that choices have consequences. You realize that investing today—in your body, in your financial future, in your family—will pay off later. So we've created an exercise program that will help you see a lifetime of gains and begin paying off immediately, and probably a lot better than your 401(k) does. You'll read about it in the next chapter.

> **HOT TIP #90**
>
> **See better in color.** Heirloom carrots in red, purple, and yellow pack more sight-protecting nutrients than the everyday orange variety.

But actually going to the gym is only part of the strategy. If you want to see the most dramatic changes in your body, it's important that you time your meals and snacks around your workouts. This simple trick will allow you to eat more calories to fuel muscle growth without gaining excess fat.

PREWORKOUT

When you eat before a workout, those calories go toward fueling your body to work optimally during your time in the gym—plus it'll improve your mood and give your the burst of energy you need to motivate you to exercise. Dutch and British researchers found that eating before your workout blunts your body's receptivity to cortisol, a fat-storing stress hormone. That speeds fat loss during your workout and for an additional 24 hours, according to scientists at Syracuse University. Just make sure to include a healthy balance of protein and carbohydrates. Eat one to two servings of carbohydrates with one serving of protein within 30 minutes before starting your workout. A great way to do this with minimal fuss? Down a protein shake.

In fact, men who eat a protein-and-carbohydrate-rich meal right before and right after their workouts build twice as much muscle as men who wait at least 5 hours to eat.

POSTWORKOUT

After your workout, consuming protein helps your body recover by providing a fresh infusion of amino acids to repair and build muscle. And carbohydrates raise your insulin levels, which slows protein breakdown and speeds muscle growth after your workout. Eat one to two servings of carbohydrates with one serving of protein 30 minutes after working out. BONUS: After you lift weights, your body's fat-storage pathways are shut off while your fat-burning mechanisms are turned on. So if you're the kind of guy who likes a cookie or a cupcake, consider this the Twinkie Hour: Now's the time to indulge. You won't use your stored protein for energy; you'll rely instead on the carbs to replenish you. And the food you eat will help you see your six-pack and also pack on lean muscle.

> **HOT TIP #91**
>
> **Step on the scale.** Do it just after you've gone to the bathroom but before you eat breakfast. Repeat every Friday. People who weigh themselves regularly are less likely to gain weight.

If you work out at lunchtime, like a lot of guys, eat one of your two snacks about 30 minutes before you work out and then go directly from the gym to the lunchroom. Rather exercise after work? Grab a snack as you're leaving the office, then eat dinner right after the gym. Work out in the mornings? Eat a light breakfast when you first get up, then chow down after you exercise. Maximum flexibility for maximum results—that's what this program is all about.

Sample *Men's Health* Diet 5-Day Meal Plan

NOTE: We'd love you to work out three times a week, preferably around lunchtime. We'd also love Blake Lively to show up at our door with a cheese pizza, a pair of Super Bowl tickets, and the

THE *MEN'S HEALTH* DIET SHOPPING LIST

FIBER-RICH GRAINS

Fresh or dried-pasta, instant oatmeal (no salt or sugar added), oats, whole-grain cereal, whole-grain bread, whole wheat flour tortillas, whole-wheat English muffins, whole-wheat pita chips, long-grain rice (brown, wild rice), quinoa

AVOCADOS, OILS, AND OTHER HEALTHY FATS

Avocados, olives, olive oil, grapeseed oil, sesame oil, canola oil, safflower oil

SPINACH, LEAFY GREENS, AND OTHER VEGETABLES

Fresh: Scallions, sprouts, beets, kale, Swiss chard, collard greens, garlic, bell peppers, romaine lettuce, celery, spinach, artichokes, asparagus, bok choy, broccoli, cabbage, carrots, cauliflower, cucumbers, green beans, leeks, mushrooms, onions, radishes
Frozen: Broccoli florets, peas

TURKEY AND OTHER LEAN MEATS

Chicken, ground beef (preferably 15% fat or less), sirloin steak, top round, pork, turkey, turkey sausage, tuna, salmon, sea bass, tilapia, trout, cod, flounder, halibut, grouper, mahi mahi, orange roughy, shrimp, scallops, lobster, crab, whey protein powder, casein protein powder

LEGUMES

Black beans, pinto beans, black-eyed peas, kidney beans, red lentils, edamame
Spreads: Peanut butter, black currant jam, black bean dip, hummus

EGGS AND DAIRY

Whole, 1%, or 2% milk; chocolate milk; yogurt; Cheddar cheese; mozzarella cheese; feta cheese; goat cheese; string-cheese sticks; ice cream; cottage cheese; omega-3 eggs

APPLES AND OTHER FRUITS

Fresh: Apples, bananas, cantaloupe, mangoes, lemons, limes, grapes, oranges, peaches, pears, melons, pineapple, tomatoes
Frozen: Blueberries, raspberries, strawberries
Dried: Raisins, prunes, apricots

NUTS AND SEEDS

Almonds, walnuts, cashews, sunflower seeds, sesame seeds, ground flaxseeds
Spreads: Almond butter, cashew butter (no salt or sugar added)

SEASONINGS

Basil, parsley, cilantro, cayenne, watercress, cumin, curry powder, chili powder, cinnamon, red-pepper flakes, reduced-sodium soy sauce, red-wine vinegar, cider vinegar deed to the Samuel Adams Brewery. But sometimes, life doesn't run that way. Maybe you need to get up early to exercise, or you can't hit the gym until the workday is through, or circumstances have conspired to make gym time a no-go for the next couple of days. Whatever your fitness dilemma, it's not a problem—again, the *Men's Health* Nutrition System is all about maximum flexibility for maximum muscle gain (and maximum fat burn). Just remember three rules:

• Always eat breakfast.

• Always eat a little something before you work out.

• Always eat a lot of something after you work out.

Wouldn't it be awesome if your girlfriend were as easygoing as this?

DAY ONE (WORKOUT DAY)

BREAKFAST: Walnut-flax oatmeal and milk

Oatmeal with chopped walnuts, ground flaxseed, bananas, and a sprinkle of cinnamon. The milk provides an instant surge of protein, and the oats keep your blood sugar in check, which regulates future cravings; the cinnamon reduces inflammation; the walnuts and flaxseeds add omega-3s and satiating healthy fat; and the bananas add heart-healthy potassium. Choose oatmeal in the form of whole oats and nothing else, such as Quaker Old Fashioned Oats.

SNACK: Protein smoothie

Chocolate whey protein powder, milk, strawberries, and bananas—the ultimate cocktail designed to have you ready for the gym. Whey is a fast-digesting protein that will prevent any stomach discomfort during exercise, while the milk, strawberries, and bananas provide the electrolyte balance that's optimal for hydration, muscle growth, and recovery.

(WORKOUT)

LUNCH: Black bean sandwich (black bean dip, olives, scallion greens, sprouts, tomatoes, and lettuce on 100 percent whole-wheat bread)

The black bean dip provides mood-boosting fiber, heart-healthy fats, and high-quality protein. The vegetables provide cancer-fighting antioxidants, bone-mass-building vitamin K, cholesterol-lowering selenium, free-radical-fighting vitamin C, and blood-pressure-lowering potassium.

SNACK: Hard-cooked eggs (2 or 3), an apple, whole-wheat bread, and strawberry jam

Hard-cooked eggs are most convenient, but it's also easy to scramble a few in the a.m. and scoop them into a microwaveable container. Don't sweat the fat: It's healthy and filling. The bread and apple will provide the carbohydrates you need to refuel after your workout and balance your potassium level to help with recovery. And the jam provides a little sugar, which will boost your insulin level so your protein is shuttled to your muscles.

DINNER: Almond beef stir-fry over brown rice with steamed kale

Stir-fry a frozen vegetable mix of your choice in a little canola oil. Then add thinly sliced grass-fed beef, a dash of reduced-sodium soy sauce, and slivered almonds. Serve over brown rice with a side of steamed kale. Starting your dinner with low-calorie, high-fiber vegetables can decrease your overall food intake by 12 percent. The beef provides high-quality lean protein plus heart-healthy omega-3s. The brown rice adds fiber, which helps stave off late-night cravings.

DAY TWO

BREAKFAST: Breakfast burrito

Scramble an egg in a little olive oil with chopped tomatoes, onions, spinach, and bell peppers, and then place the mixture in a whole-wheat flour tortilla. Top with a sprinkling of shredded Cheddar cheese.

SNACK: Whole-wheat toast with almond spread and apples

LUNCH: Ultimate tuna salad

Combine red leaf lettuce, spinach, chunk light tuna (water-packed), grape tomatoes, navy beans, Cheddar cheese, carrots, broccoli, red bell peppers, ground flaxseed, and sesame seeds. Dress with olive oil and balsamic vinegar.

SNACK: Greek yogurt

Greek-style yogurt is a lifter's dream: It's easy to carry and packed with protein. Skip yogurts with fruit and sugar; to add flavor, drop in a few berries or nuts.

HOT TIP #92

Try a lusty fruit. Lychees pack magnesium, which boosts circulation to the pelvic region.

DINNER: Red lentil burritos

Sauté onions, broccoli, carrots, tomato sauce, curry powder, cumin, and chili powder. Add cooked red lentils and sun-dried tomatoes. Serve in whole-wheat tortillas with Cheddar cheese, yogurt, and chopped cilantro. Eat with a side salad of fresh baby spinach mixed with olive oil and grated Romano cheese.

DAY THREE (WORKOUT DAY)

BREAKFAST: Whole-grain cereal, toast with almond butter and chopped dried apricots, and a glass of milk

SNACK: Cottage cheese, oatmeal, and an apple

Cottage cheese contains all of the benefits of a protein shake without the blending. It's a high-quality source of protein that will also help you lose weight because of its high amount of calcium. The oatmeal and apple will boost your energy so you can lift heavier weights and curb hunger during your workout.

(WORKOUT)

LUNCH: Indonesian chicken salad sandwich

Mix peanut butter, a dash of water, white wine vinegar, minced garlic, and red-pepper flakes with strips of organic chicken, kale, and onion. Spread on whole-wheat bread.

SNACK: Two cups (16 ounces) of chocolate milk

Refresh and rebuild at the same time. A study in the *Journal of the American College of Nutrition* shows that chocolate milk may be the ideal postworkout beverage for building muscle.

DINNER: Seared wild salmon with mango chutney, eggplant, and Swiss chard

Marinate the salmon in a mixture of lemon juice, paprika, salt, and pepper and then sear it in a little olive oil. On top, add a mixture of finely chopped mango, bell pepper, onion, lime juice, mint, and jalapeño pepper. Serve with a side of grilled eggplant and steamed Swiss chard. (Note: We strongly recommend wild salmon over the farm-raised type; wild salmon has a much more favorable omega-3 profile, and is much lower in obesity-promoting pesticides. All "Atlantic salmon" are farm-raised. Choose wild Alaskan salmon instead.)

DAY FOUR

BREAKFAST: Berry-banana smoothie

Combine frozen blueberries, raspberries, and a banana (fresh or frozen) in a blender with yogurt. Add some 1% milk and peanut butter. Blend until smooth. Serve with a whole-grain English muffin with black currant jam.

SNACK: Fried egg and cheese sandwich

The egg provides satiating protein to help you power through your day.

LUNCH: Free-range chicken salad

Combine cooked free-range organic chicken, spinach, apples, and almonds, and mix with a bit of yogurt, Dijon mustard, and celery.

SNACK: Banana and peanut butter

DINNER: Buffalo burger on a whole-wheat bun topped with baked and mashed garnet yams, sautéed onions, and roasted red peppers. Serve with a steamed-spinach salad.

DAY FIVE (WORKOUT DAY)

BREAKFAST: Spinach omelet with yogurt and blueberries

Chop a bunch of spinach and sauté it in a little olive oil. Stir together 1 egg and a bit more chopped spinach, pour it over the sautéed spinach, and cook until the egg is set. The yogurt provides probiotics, which support weight loss, digestion, and healthy immune functioning. The blueberries add antioxidants, which studies suggest can help prevent cancer, diabetes, and age-related memory loss.

SNACK: Whey powder mixed with two servings of berries

This milk-derived product continues to rule the gym. Mix it with milk instead of water if you want a bit more protein. The added fruit not only improves taste, but also offers sustained energy.

(WORKOUT)

LUNCH: Split-pea soup with spelt crackers and a fresh baby spinach side salad

SNACK: Chicken, turkey, or tuna wrap

Toss one of these standbys in a whole-wheat wrap and add lettuce and tomatoes for the ultimate postworkout meal. Have a serving of ice cream for dessert, which provides the small dose of sugar that fuels muscle growth.

DINNER: Almond rainbow trout with watercress

Pan-fry farm-raised rainbow trout in almond oil with sliced raw almonds. Top with cider vinegar and watercress. Serve with a side of collard greens sautéed in olive oil and garlic.

Eating fat won't make you fat any more than eating money will make you rich.

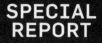

WHAT'S IN MACGYVER'S FRIDGE? 24 SMART FOOD FIXES THAT WILL SMOOTH OVER EVERYTHING FROM BIG-MEETING JITTERS TO BIG-DATE ANGST.

Wouldn't it be great if you could make your enemies lose consciousness just by tweaking their necks, like Mr. Spock? Or break down any alibi by playing with your opponent's mind, like detective Robert Goren on *Law and Order: Criminal Intent*? Or turn a rusted bucket of bolts into a high-performance vehicle, like Murdock

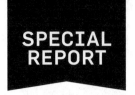

from *The A-Team*? Or defuse a bomb with nothing more than a paper clip, a ballpoint pen, and a pair of tube socks, like MacGyver?

Well, you might not be able to stop crime, save a hostage, or reverse the future of the universe, but you can defuse some annoying day-to-day problems with a little MacGyver-like ingenuity and a well-stocked pantry. Dull shoes before a big meeting? Eat a banana, then use the inside of the peel to shine up your dogs. No shaving cream? Peanut butter will do in a pinch (but it's pretty gross). Girlfriend's cat scratched your new leather briefcase? Dab a little olive oil on to cover up the mark. (It's up to you to figure out a way to cover up the cat's mysterious disappearance.) Slugs eating your tomato plants? A platter of beer will drown them—plus they'll die happy.

But sometimes the enemy isn't a lost dopp kit, a disagreeable kitten, or an invasion of mollusks. Sometimes, the enemy is within—a body (and mind) that's just not performing up to snuff. Fortunately, food is also your best weapon when it comes to priming your body for battle—whether your adversary is chronic stress, nagging aches and pains, or just a case of the heebie-jeebies. All you need to ask is WWME: What would MacGyver eat?

> **HOT TIP #93**
>
> **Wake up to water.**
> Drink at least
> 16 ounces of chilled
> H2O as soon as
> you rise. German
> scientists found this
> boosts metabolism
> by 24 percent for
> 90 minutes after-
> ward. (A smaller
> amount of water
> had no effect.)
> A general rule of
> thumb: Guzzle
> at least a gallon
> of water a day.

When . . . you're facing a big day at work
Bacon or ham and fried eggs

The protein in this power meal will keep you feeling full throughout the morning. A University of Illinois study found that people who eat more protein and less carbs than are usually in conventional diet-plan meals find it easier to stick to a diet. Protein is satiating, to power you through the day, and may also boost calorie burn, the study authors say. Plus, when you digest eggs, protein fragments are produced that can prevent your blood vessels from narrowing—which may help keep your blood pressure from rising. In fact, Canadian scientists found in a lab study that the hotter the eggs, the more potent the proteins, and frying them sends their temps soaring.

When . . . you're caught in stop-and-go traffic
Sugar-free chewing gum

In a British study, people who chewed gum while taking math, memory, and concentration tests reported an average 13 percent drop in stress. The study authors believe that the act of chewing might lead to subconscious associations with positive social settings (like mealtimes), which may reduce tension. Sugar-free gum has the additional benefit of knocking off bacteria, which can multiply in your pie hole when you're stressed or dehydrated.

When . . . you look in the mirror and notice another wrinkle and spin into a dark crisis of the soul while Aerosmith's "Dream On" is playing in the background . . .
Guacamole

A study in the *Journal of the American College of Nutrition* found that people with high intakes of olive oil showed fewer wrinkles than those with high intakes of butter. The reason: monounsaturated fats, which are found in abundance in olive oil. Drizzle some on your salad, but if that's not convenient, grab a side of guacamole—

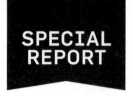

avocados have the same monounsaturated fats as olive oil, plus plenty of fiber and healthy B vitamins.

When . . . you dropped your toothbrush in the toilet
Monterey Jack

Researchers found that eating less than a quarter ounce of Jack, Cheddar, Gouda, or mozzarella cheese boosts your saliva pH level to protect your pearly whites from cavities.

When . . . you need to . . . to . . . focus
Peppermint tea

Researchers in Cincinnati found that periodic whiffs of peppermint increase people's concentration and performance on tasks requiring sustained attention. (Sniff: "I can do this.") Now, we know most guys don't keep peppermint tea in their desks. But think of it as a scientific improvement over the alternative: British researchers discovered that sleepy people who downed a sugary, caffeinated drink like soda had slower reaction times and more lapses in attention after 80 minutes than people who drank a sugar-free beverage.

When . . . your CEO has the oratory restraint of Fidel Castro, and he's just invited you to an afternoon-long meeting
Grilled salmon with spinach and carrots

This meal is scientifically proven to prevent doodling and drooling—the two potentially career-crushing side effects of soporific assemblies. Stay awake effortlessly by grabbing a seafaring sidekick. Salmon contains tyrosine, an amino acid that your brain uses to make dopamine and norepinephrine—neurochemicals that keep you alert. The brain-balm omega-3s in salmon may also help tame your neurotic tendencies. Halibut and trout are good alternatives to salmon. And leafy greens provide the B vitamin folate, used by the brain to make the mood controllers serotonin, dopamine, and nor-epinephrine. Folate shortages have been linked to depression. Add carrots: Beta-carotene may help reduce the effects of oxidative stress on your memory.

When . . . you're feeling the sniffles coming on
Ginseng

In a Canadian study, people who took 400 milligrams of ginseng extract a day had 56 percent fewer recurring colds than those who popped placebos. Studies suggest ginseng can boost the activity of key immune cells. Another benefit: Ginseng might boost your brainpower. British researchers found that people who swallowed 200 milli-grams of the extract an hour before tak-ing a cognitive test scored significantly better than when they skipped the supplement.

AND THIS: Eat kiwi fruits, oranges, and red bell peppers. All three are packed with vitamin C. Studies suggest that tak-ing in at least 200 milligrams daily may help shorten the duration of your symp-toms the next time you're under the weather.

> **HOT TIP #94**
>
> **Zap the TV commercials.**
> Foods advertised on television are usually loaded with sugar and fat. Research in the *Journal of the American Dietetic Association* reveals that a 2,000-calorie diet of such foods would exceed the RDA for sugar by 25 times and the RDA for fat by 20 times. Deflect those cues with dark-chocolate.

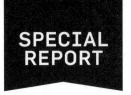

When...you've got a bad cough
Honey

Penn State scientists found that honey is better at lessening cough frequency and severity than dextromethorphan, the most common active ingredient in over-the-counter cough meds.

When...you can't stop hiccupping
Sugar

A study published in the *New England Journal of Medicine* found that 1 teaspoon of table sugar, swallowed dry, cured hiccups in 95 percent of people—some of whom had been hiccupping as long as 6 weeks.

When...it sounds like someone has snuck a whoopie cushion under your chair...except there's no whoopie cushion
Sauerkraut

A study published in the *European Journal of Gastroenterology and Hepatology* found that *Lactobacillus plantarum* 299V, the bacterium used to ferment foods like sauerkraut, relieved gas symptoms in 33 of 40 people studied. (*Men's Health* editors read this kind of stuff all the time, so you don't have to.)

When...you're gearing up for an intense workout
Green tea

In a 2009 report from the American Society for Nutrition, scientists revealed that exercisers who drank green tea lost twice as much weight and had the greatest declines in total abdominal fat.

When . . . you're gearing up for an intense workout and the pollen count is through the roof
Pink grapefruit

Pink grapefruit is rich in two compounds: lycopene, which has been shown to decrease symptoms of wheezing, asthma, and shortness of breath in people when they exercise; and beta-cryptoxanthin, which helps decrease inflammation in the joints and may improve the function of the respiratory system.

When . . . you just finished an intense workout
Coffee

University of Georgia scientists reported that taking a caffeine supplement (equal to 2 cups of coffee) after exercise reduces muscle soreness more than pain relievers can. Caffeine blocks a chemical that activates pain receptors.

When . . . you just finished an intense workout and now you want a reward, damn it!
Beer

Researchers at Granada University in Spain have discovered that the combination of sugars, salts, and bubbles in beer help people absorb fluids more quickly. This may just be an excuse, but as excuses go, it's a good one!

HOT TIP #95

Go for the D-cup. A vitamin D deficiency can make it harder for you to lose weight, a University of Minnesota study reveals. Milk is your best dietary source of vitamin D. In another study, dieters who downed five servings of dairy a day lost more abdominal fat than those who had just three.

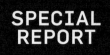

When . . . Uncle Teddy is dragging you to the all-you-can-eat buffet
An apple

Discipline ain't easy when second helpings are free. But in a study at Penn State, researchers found that those who ate an apple 15 minutes before lunch consumed 15 percent fewer calories than those who drank apple juice, ate applesauce, or had nothing at all.

When . . . you notice a few new gray hairs
Pinot noir

As elixirs of youth go, wine has its pros and cons. University of Toronto researchers discovered that one alcoholic drink causes people's blood vessels to relax—but the second drink begins to reverse the effect. You'll be even more relaxed knowing that that glass of red contains resveratrol, an antioxidant linked to everything from cancer prevention to heart-disease protection. And pinot noirs generally have the highest concentrations of the compound. But again, this isn't a license to swill. A small 2007 study found people with alcohol or drug problems were twice as likely to have prematurely gray hair as those without substance-abuse issues. Long-term abuse may speed aging and the loss of melanocytes, cells that give hair its pigment.

HOT TIP #96

Get up, stand up. Americans sit 8 percent more than they did in 1980. Studies show that the more time you spend sitting, the greater your risk of heart attack, regardless of how fit you are. And standing for three 10-minute phone calls a day will burn an extra 33 calories. That's 2 pounds gone every year!

When . . . you're on a hot date
Oysters for an appetizer, steak for an entrée, and dark chocolate for dessert

Protein can boost levels of brain chemicals that heighten arousal. Oysters and steak also contain zinc, which may help maintain the testosterone level. And two forms of an amino acid in oysters have been linked to testosterone production in rats, but it's unclear whether oysters have any true libido-boosting influence. Go for the suggestive effect. As for the chocolate? A woman becomes more aroused from dark chocolate melting in her mouth than from kissing, British scientists found. The chocolate not only raises her heart rate, but brain-wave monitoring shows it also makes her more relaxed and alert.

A CAVEAT: White chocolate won't do the trick. Since it has no cocoa solids, it lacks the methylxanthines (caffeine and theobromine) found in dark and milk chocolates. These stimulants can make you feel more energetic and alert, and cocoa solids also have the heart-healthy antioxidants that make darker chocolates so appealing to your cardiologist.

When . . . you're in the mood, she's in the mood, and you want to make a baby
Brazil nuts and strawberries

Cigarette smoke, air pollution, and other toxins in the air can damage sperm, altering the DNA inside the cells and leading to fertility issues. Brazil nuts are a top source of selenium, a mineral that boosts sperm health while also helping your swimmers achieve more Phelpsian levels. Strawberries are great sources of vitamin C. University of Texas researchers found that men who consumed at least 200 milligrams of vitamin C a day had higher sperm counts than men who took in less.

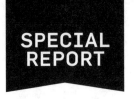
When . . . life feels like it has no meaning
Flaxseed

Flax is the best known source of alpha-linolenic acid—a healthy fat that improves the workings of the cerebral cortex, the area of the brain that processes sensory information, including that of pleasure. To meet your quota, sprinkle it into smoothies or on salads, or make it the secret ingredient in a PB&J.

When . . . you're on a hot date and you realize she's a lot smarter than you are
Blueberries

Researchers at Tufts University have found that blueberries and the anthocyanins they contain may make brain cells respond better to incoming messages and might even spur the growth of new nerve cells. This may take longer than just eating a dessert, though.

When . . . you're on a hot date and you realize you have garlic breath
Milk

A study from Ohio State, published in the *Journal of Food Science*, found that the combination of water, fat, and sodium caseinate in milk could help reduce concentrations of volatile compounds responsible for foul-smelling garlic breath.

When . . . you had such an awesome day that you just can't fall asleep
Oatmeal with sliced bananas and walnuts

Sleep is inspired by the hormone melatonin, but stress or excitement can disrupt melatonin's release. Bring your brain back down to earth by whipping up a bowl of instant oatmeal and topping it with sliced bananas and crushed walnuts, both rich in melatonin.

What won't do the trick: warm milk. Contrary to popular belief, warm milk will keep you up, not knock you out. Blame the protein in the milk, which can reduce serotonin levels and delay the onset of sleep.

When . . . you want to prevent a hangover
A virgin screwdriver

For last call, go with a girly drink. Fructose, one of the sugars in orange juice, can speed the metabolism of alcohol by as much as 25 percent. Vitamin C also helps combat binge-related cell damage.

When . . . you wake up the next morning and realize you forgot to prevent the hangover
Gatorade and toast with jam

Your most important play is to replace fluids and electrolytes lost by sweating, urinating, crying, or whatever other bodily embarrassment you might have been experiencing the night before. A sports beverage will help replace these faster, while the fructose in the jam will help speed the metabolization of the alcohol and the toast will just steady your stomach some.

please save the date to celebrate with us

sunday evening, june 19, north bank park

blocks of hotel rooms available at:
- hyatt on capitol square, 614-228-1234
- doubletree guest suites, 614-228-4600

details: www.northbankwedding.tumblr.com

more to come...

rachel scott and aaron wasserman
114 willow street, apt. 3
cambridge, ma 02141

BOSTON MA USA

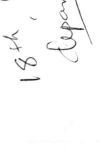

Mr. Mark Owen
2 Happy Hollow Road
Wayland, MA 01778

18th, 19th
aaron 2011

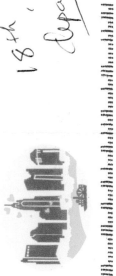

1774+3504

rachel and aaron are getting married!

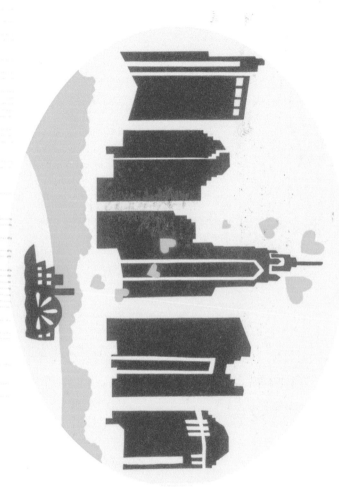

sunday, june 19, 2011 • columbus, ohio

8

THE *MEN'S HEALTH* MUSCLE SYSTEM
THE GREATEST WORKOUT YOU'LL EVER GET—INSIDE A GYM OR OUT.

Walking into the gym and expecting a great workout is like walking into the supermarket and expecting a gourmet meal. The basic ingredients are there, but like they say in the infomercials, results may vary. With working out, as with cooking, a little bit of smarts, dedication, creativity, and knowledge will make all the difference between perfect prime rib and warmed-over gristle.

In fact, your best chance at a great workout might come from avoiding the gym—or at least the advice and equipment there—altogether. Why? Because the run-of-the-mill fitness club already has three strikes against it.

STRIKE ONE: The trainers

There are nearly 200,000 fitness trainers at work in the United States, doing the kind of stuff that's traditionally been the province of medical professionals—giving out nutritional advice; testing our cardiovascular, muscular, and nervous systems; and jacking up our heart rates and blood pressure with prescriptive programs. And what kind of training do these exercise experts have? In most cases, little or none. There's absolutely no governing body or set of standardized tests that anyone has to pass before coming to your gym or your house and starting to make you sweat. So while there are plenty of great trainers out there, telling the gamers from the goofballs takes a little research.

Now, you might be thinking, "At my gym, they have 'certified personal trainers.'" Sure, most gyms like their trainers to be certified, but by whom? There are close to 300 certifications available in the United States, many of them meaningless. (Want certification as a Group Fitness Instructor from the American Fitness Professionals and Associates? Just send $385 to a PO box in Ship Bottom, New Jersey, and you'll get two textbooks and some DVDs that tell you everything you need to know. You never even have to meet with anyone. Just pass a simple test—you get to take it over and over again until you do—and you're certified!) Only two certifying bodies are really worth their salt: the National Strength and Conditioning Association (which grants the prestigious Certified Strength and Conditioning Specialist degree, or CSCS) and the American College of Sports Medicine.

That said, there are plenty of personal trainers who know what they're doing and can help you make a big difference in your condition. And hiring a personal trainer does have one solid benefit, regardless of his or her skill: You're paying for the trainer's time, and that alone may help you stick with a workout. Still, if you want to hire a teammate in your quest for fitness, make sure you grill the person the way you would any potential employee. (A good starting place is our set of questions on page 190.)

STRIKE TWO: The equipment

Most gyms have rows and rows of shiny, newfangled weight machines that duplicate the movements found in free-weight workouts. They have chest press machines, shoulder press machines, even something called a Smith machine, which offers guided movement on exercises like the squat. The exercise you should be doing on machines like these? Walk aways. Here's how you do them: You look at the machine, and then you walk away.

There are two reasons why. First, studies show that you simply get a better workout using free weights. Take for instance the leg extension machine. University of Kentucky researchers studied 23 patients with knee pain to see what made them stronger—using a simple set of stairs or using one of these machines. They found that in every measure of leg strength, simple stepups using a flight of stairs built strength more effectively. The leg extension machine didn't make test subjects stronger at any tasks, except one: using the leg extension machine. It did nothing for their functioning in the real world. Another study in the *Journal of Strength and Conditioning Research* found that men who did squats using free weights activated 43 percent more muscle than men performing squats on the Smith machine.

Second, machines may seem safer, but they can lead to injury because they lock our bodies into planes of movement that aren't natural. For example, when you walk or climb a set of stairs or squat a light weight, your thighbone rotates under your kneecap—the normal movement of your lower body. But on a leg-extension machine, your kneecap rotates instead. That puts a lot of strain on the knee ligaments and patella, the soft padding under the kneecap.

So if exercise machines are both ineffective and dangerous, why are gyms so packed with them? Simple: Because they want you to think you can't get a great workout without all that fancy equipment, so you'll have to keep coming back to the gym! The *Men's Health* Muscle System, on the other hand, requires only a single set of dumbbells, and you don't even need a gym. You can perform it in your living room, basement, garage, prison cell, high school auditorium, two-seater outhouse, or any other facility you might have access to.

You can, by the way, also do it at your local fitness club. (And if you do happen to swing by the gym, first familiarize yourself with our list of exercise machines you should never, ever use, on page 186.)

STRIKE THREE: The spandex.

Or more specifically, the pretty young things squeezed into the spandex. Every moment you spend standing around waiting for the bench press or a cable station—or, let's face it, chatting up a prospective date—is less time you're spending challenging your muscles and igniting your metabolism. More sitting around means less intensity, and that undercuts your ability to make quick gains from your time in the gym. And with less time than ever to exercise, you need a workout that guarantees results, fast.

That's why *Men's Health* has designed this fat-burning, muscle-building workout with minimum equipment requirements and maximum efficiency in mind: 10 exercises performed as a high-intensity circuit that works every muscle in your body.

But this isn't your traditional program filled with the routine

3 sets of 10 reps. Those are arbitrary goals set by some gym teacher back in sixth grade. This plan works based on time—the ultimate motivator—and it allows you to challenge your body and push your fitness to new levels. Instead of worrying about a goal number of reps, each set is timed so you can push yourself to reach a new personal record with each workout. This approach allows you to choose if you want to perform more reps or add more weight, putting you in control of your goals. You'll be changing your body, strengthening your heart, and doing everything you need to supercharge your metabolism and look and live healthier than ever.

Directions

Do this circuit 3 days a week. Perform 1 set of each exercise in succession. Each set consists of doing the exercise as many times as you can in 30 seconds. Use only perfect form—it doesn't count if you cheat, Mr. McGwire—and when your 30 seconds are up, give yourself 15 seconds to rest before moving on to the next exercise. Rest for 2 minutes after you've completed the entire sequence. Then repeat the whole process two more times for a total of 3 circuits per workout.

If you get tired and can't continue exercising for the entire 30 seconds, stop and rest for a few seconds, and then resume performing reps until the time is up. For each exercise, you should start with a weight that you can use for 10 to 12 perfect reps.

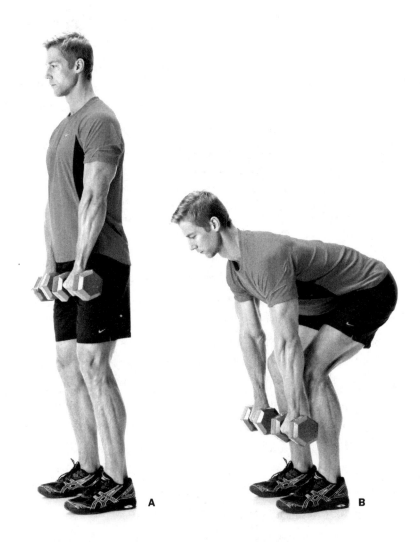

A **B**

Dumbbell straight-leg deadlift

Grab a pair of dumbbells with an overhand grip and hold them in front of your thighs, arms hanging straight down. Stand with your feet hip-width apart and your knees slightly bent **(A)**. Without changing the bend in your knees, bend at your hips and lower your torso until it's almost parallel to the floor **(B)**. Pause, then raise your torso back to the starting position.

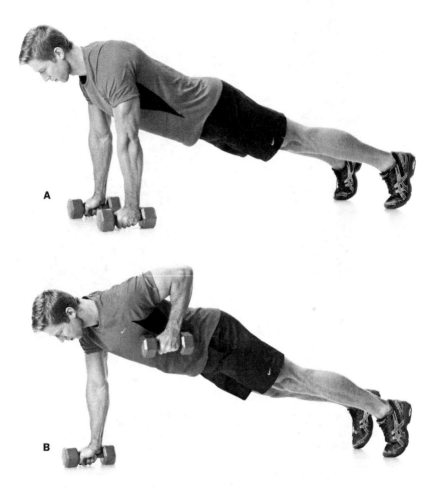

Dumbbell plank and row

Grab a pair of hex dumbbells with an overhand grip and assume a pushup position, your arms straight (**A**). Keeping your core stiff, balance your weight on your left arm as you pull the dumbbell in your right hand up to the side of your chest, bending your arm as you pull it upward (**B**). Pause, and then quickly lower the dumbbell. Repeat with your left arm.

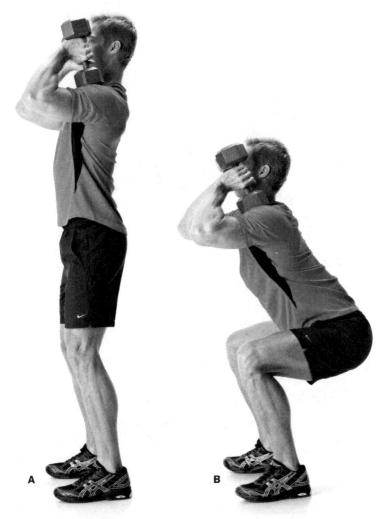

A   B

Dumbbell front squat

Stand and hold a pair of dumbbells so that your palms are facing
each other and a dumbbell head is resting on the meatiest part of
each shoulder (**A**). Keep your body as upright as you can at all times.
Brace your abs and lower your body as far as you can by pushing
your hips back and bending your knees (**B**). Don't allow your elbows
to drop down as you squat. Pause, then push yourself back to the
starting position.

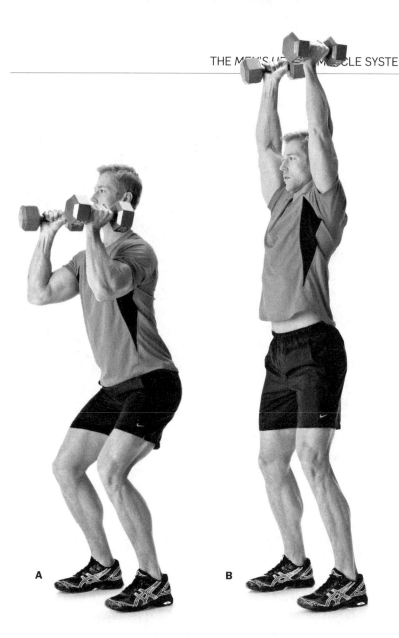

A   B

Dumbbell push press

Stand and hold a pair of dumbbells so that your palms are facing
each other and the dumbbells are parallel to the floor (**A**). Keep
your body upright as you bend slightly at the knees, then explosively push up with your legs as you press the dumbbells over your
head (**B**). Pause, then lower the weights to the starting position.

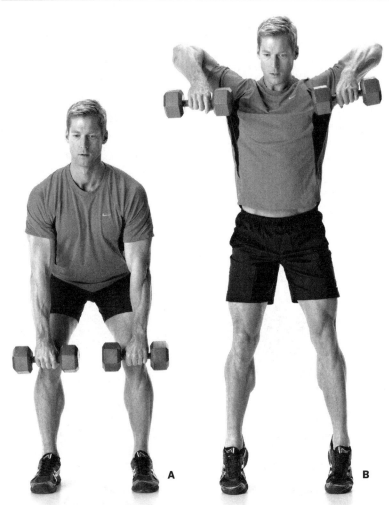

A   B

Dumbbell high pull

Hold a pair of dumbbells just below the fronts of your knees with your palms facing your legs, your hips pushed back, and your knees slightly bent (**A**). With your back flat and arms straight, pull both dumbbells upward as fast as you can by thrusting your hips forward and explosively standing up (**B**). Keep the dumbbells as close to your body as possible and bring them up to shoulder height. (At the top of the movement, your elbows should angle out like you're doing the funky chicken.) Return to the starting position.

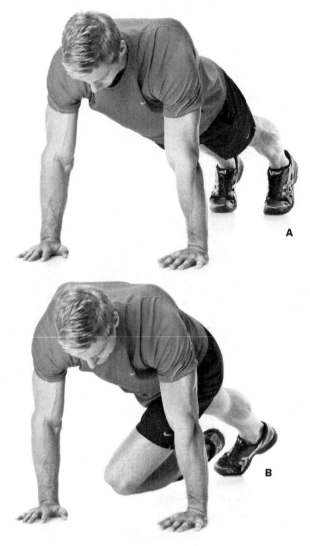

Cross-body mountain climber

Assume a pushup position with your arms completely straight (**A**). Lift your right foot off the floor, then bend your right knee and bring it up under your body, toward your left elbow, without changing the arch in your lower back (**B**). Lower your leg back to the starting position. Then raise your left foot off the ground and bring your left knee to your right elbow. Alternate back and forth until time is up.

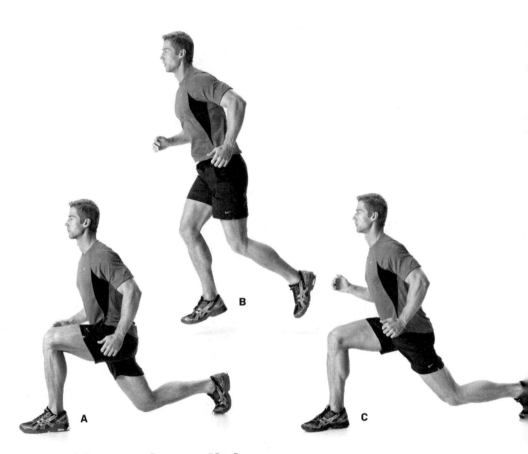

Alternating split jump

Stand in a staggered stance with your feet 2 to 3 feet apart, your left foot in front of your right. Keeping your torso upright, bend your legs and lower your body into a lunge position (**A**). At the bottom of the movement, your left thigh should be parallel to the ground, and your right thigh should be perpendicular to the ground. Now jump with enough force to propel both feet off the floor (**B**). While you're in the air, scissor-kick your legs so you land with your right leg forward and your left leg behind you (**C**). Repeat, alternating your forward leg for the duration of the set.

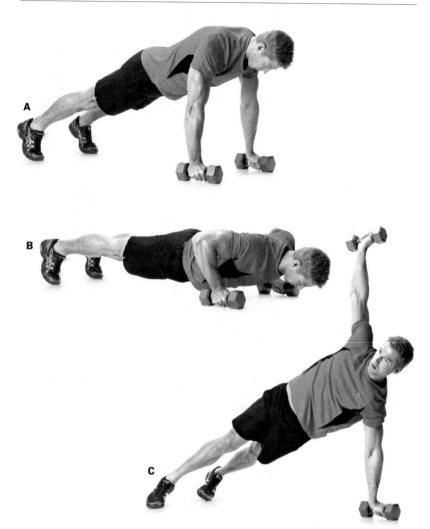

T-pushup

Grab a pair of hex dumbbells with an overhand grip and assume a pushup position, your arms straight (**A**). Bend your elbows and lower your body until your chest nearly touches the floor (**B**). As you push yourself back up, lift your right hand and rotate the right side of your body as you raise the dumbbell straight up over your shoulder until your body forms a T (**C**). Reverse the move and repeat, this time rotating your left side.

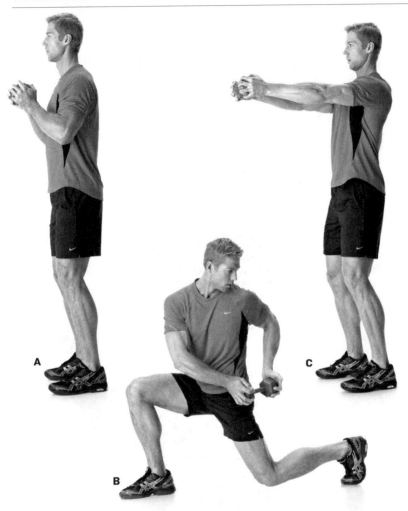

A **B** **C**

Reverse lunge and swing

Grasp the head of a dumbbell with both hands and hold the weight hanging down in front of your chest with your arms bent (**A**). Step backward with your left leg and bend your left knee until it almost touches the floor. As you step back, rotate your shoulders and swing the dumbbell to the outside of your left hip (**B**). Press back up to the starting position and swing the dumbbell to eye level with your arms extended (**C**). Return the dumbbell to the starting position and repeat on your other side.

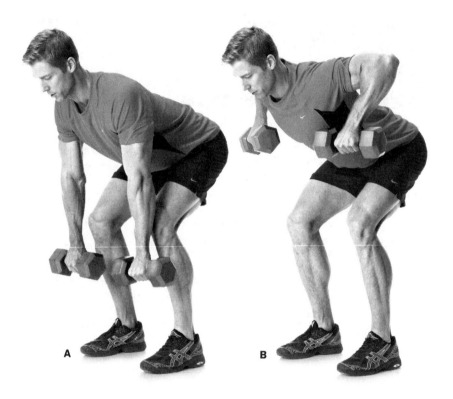

A   **B**

Dumbbell row

Grab a pair of dumbbells, bend at your hips (don't round your lower back), and lower your torso until it's nearly parallel to the floor. Let the dumbbells hang at arm's length, palms inward (**A**). Without moving your torso, row the weights upward by raising your upper arms, bending your elbows, and squeezing your shoulder blades together (**B**). Keep the dumbbells close to the side of your body at the top of the movement. Pause, lower the dumbbells, and repeat.

THE 10 EXERCISE MACHINES YOU MUST AVOID

For this list of no-no exercises, we consulted Stuart McGill, PhD, professor of spine biomechanics at the University of Waterloo in Ontario; Nicholas DiNubile, MD, an orthopedic surgeon and author of *FrameWork: Your 7-Step Program for Healthy Muscles, Bones, and Joints*; and trainer Vern Gambetta, author of *Athletic Development: The Art and Science of Functional Sports Conditioning*.

1. Seated Leg Extension

WHAT IT'S SUPPOSED TO DO: Train the quadriceps

WHAT IT ACTUALLY DOES: It strengthens a motion your legs aren't actually designed to do and can put undue strain on the ligaments and tendons surrounding the kneecaps.

A BETTER EXERCISE: One-legged body-weight squats. Stand with your feet shoulder-width apart. Lift one leg up and bend the opposite knee, dipping down as far as you can with control while flexing at the hip, knee, and ankle. Use a rail for support until you develop the requisite leg strength and balance. Aim for 5 to 10 reps on each leg. (If you are susceptible to knee pain, do the Bulgarian split squat instead, resting the top of one foot on a bench positioned 2 to 3 feet behind you. Descend until your thigh is parallel to the floor and then stand back up. Do 5 to 10 reps per leg.)

2.
Seated Military Press

WHAT IT'S SUPPOSED TO DO: Train the shoulders and triceps

WHAT IT ACTUALLY DOES: Overhead pressing can put shoulder joints in vulnerable biomechanical positions. It puts undue stress on the shoulders, and the movement doesn't let you use your hips to assist your shoulders, which is the natural way to push something overhead.

A BETTER EXERCISE: Medicine-ball throws. Stand 3 feet from a concrete wall. Bounce a rubber medicine ball off a spot on the wall 4 feet above your head, squatting to catch the ball and rising to throw it upward in one continuous motion. Aim for 15 to 20 reps. Alternative: Standing alternate dumbbell presses. Stand with your feet shoulder-width apart, elbows bent, and a dumbbell in each hand at shoulder height, palms facing out. As you push the right dumbbell overhead, shift the right hip forward. Lower the weight, then switch to the left side.

3.
Seated Lat Pull-Down (Behind the Neck)

WHAT IT'S SUPPOSED TO DO: Train lats, upper back, and biceps

WHAT IT ACTUALLY DOES: Unless you have very flexible shoulders, it's difficult to do correctly, so it can cause pinching in the shoulder joint and damage the rotator cuff.

A BETTER EXERCISE: Incline pullups. Place a bar in the squat rack at waist height, grab the bar with both hands, and hang from the bar with your legs stretched out in front of you. Keep your torso stiff and pull your chest to the bar 10 to 15 times. To make it harder, lower the bar; to make it easier, raise the bar.

4.
Seated Pec Deck

WHAT IT'S SUPPOSED TO DO: Train the chest and shoulders

WHAT IT ACTUALLY DOES: It can put the shoulder in an unstable position and place excessive stress on the shoulder joint and its connective tissue.

A BETTER EXERCISE: Incline pushups. Get into a pushup position on the floor, but with your feet resting on a bench. Aim for 15 to 20 reps. If this is too easy, progress to regular pushups and plyometric pushups (where you push up with enough force that your hands come off the ground), and aim for 5 to 8 reps.

5.
Seated Hip Abductor Machine

WHAT IT'S SUPPOSED TO DO: Train the outer thighs

WHAT IT ACTUALLY DOES: Because you are seated, it trains a movement that has no functional use. If done with excessive weight and jerky technique, it can put undue pressure on the spine.

A BETTER EXERCISE: Loop a heavy, short resistance band around your legs (at your ankles). Sidestep out 20 paces and back with control. This is much harder than it sounds.

6.
Seated Rotation Machine

WHAT IT'S SUPPOSED TO DO: Train the abdominals and obliques

WHAT IT ACTUALLY DOES: Because the pelvis doesn't move with the chest, this exercise can put excessive twisting forces on the spine.

A BETTER EXERCISE: Do the cable wood chop. Attach a rope handle to the high pulley of a cable station. Stand with your feet shoulder-width apart and your right side facing the weight stack. Rotate your body to grip the rope with both hands. Your torso should be turned toward the cable machine. In one movement, pull the rope down and past your left hip as you simultaneously rotate your torso (your right foot should pivot). Reverse the movement to return to the starting position. Aim for 10 to 12 reps, switch sides, and repeat.

7.
Seated Leg Press

WHAT IT'S SUPPOSED TO DO: Train the quadriceps, glutes, and hamstrings

WHAT IT ACTUALLY DOES: It often forces the spine to flex without engaging any of the necessary stabilization muscles of the hips, glutes, shoulders, and lower back.

A BETTER EXERCISE: Body-weight squats. Stand with your feet shoulder-width apart, arms at your sides. Now squat down as if sitting in a low chair, while reaching your arms straight out in front of you for balance. Focus on descending with control as far as you can without rounding your lower back or letting your knees drift inward. Aim for 15 to 20 for a set, and increase the number of sets as you develop strength.

8.
Smith Machine Squats

WHAT IT'S SUPPOSED TO DO: Train the chest, biceps, and legs

WHAT IT ACTUALLY DOES: The alignment of the machine—the bar is attached to a vertical sliding track—makes for linear, not natural, arched movements. This puts stress on the knees, shoulders, and lower back.

A BETTER EXERCISE: Body-weight squats. See "Seated Leg Press" for instructions.

9.
Roman Chair Back Extension

WHAT IT'S SUPPOSED TO DO: Train the spinal erectors

WHAT IT ACTUALLY DOES: Repeatedly flexing the back while it's supporting weight places pressure on the spine and increases the risk of damaging your disks.

A BETTER EXERCISE: The bird dog. Crouch on all fours and extend your right arm forward and your left leg backward. Hold for 7 seconds. Do 10 reps and then switch to the opposite side.

10.
Roman Chair Situp

WHAT IT'S SUPPOSED TO DO: Train the abdominals and hip flexors

WHAT IT ACTUALLY DOES: The crunching motion can put undue stress on the lower back when it is in a vulnerable rounded position.

A BETTER EXERCISE: The plank. Lie facedown on the floor. Prop yourself up on your forearms, palms down. Rise up on your toes. Keep your back flat and contract your glutes, abdominals, and lats to keep your butt from sticking up. Hold this pose for 20 to 60 seconds.

BONUS: **HOW TO FIND A PERSONAL TRAINER**

Even if you love the *Men's Health* Muscle System—and we know you will—sometimes hiring a trainer to put you through the paces is the extra motivation you need to help you stick to a routine. Certifications are important (you want some education), but anyone can study for a test and pass it. Fitness groups like the National Strength and Conditioning Association and the American College of Sports Medicine offer credible testing programs.

But if you really want to make sure you're hiring someone who knows what he or she is doing, you need to conduct a killer interrogation. We went to Alwyn Cosgrove, co-owner of Results Fitness in Santa Clarita, California, and Mike Boyle, owner of Mike Boyle Strength and Conditioning in Woburn and North Andover, Massachusetts—they're two of the brightest fitness minds at two of the best gyms in the world. They shared exactly what they look for when they hire new staff members, which is what you need to know before you spend your money on hired help. Here are the things you should evaluate when you go searching for a trainer.

1) DO THEY EVALUATE YOU FIRST?

A trainer can't take you to where you want to go until he or she knows where you're starting from. There are different ways that a trainer can evaluate your body, but you need to be active during the process. No trainer should ever write a program without seeing how you move and assessing your weaknesses. Remember, the benefit of having a trainer is that you receive personalized feedback designed for you.

2) HOW GOOD IS HIS OR HER PROGRAM?

You don't need an advanced degree in order to find this out. Here are three signs that your trainer has developed a good program.

A) LENGTH OF TIME. A program should consider both your short- and long-term goals.

But trainers worth their salt should have a vision of how to address your flaws and design a program that lasts for a decent length of time. That doesn't mean you shouldn't see results fast. In fact, you should begin seeing changes in only a few weeks. But you want your trainer to provide a plan that goes beyond those initial changes and helps you stay healthy for good.

B) CONSISTENCY. A trainer who changes the workout every single time is not allowing you to adapt and improve. As you'll experience with the *Men's Health* Muscle System, you need to have a set program that will allow your body to adapt as you become stronger and lose more body fat. It may seem beneficial to change exercises every day, but that will actually prevent you from seeing rapid changes in fat loss and muscle gain. Also, if you make changes every time, you'll never know what works.

C) PROGRESSION. Just because your program doesn't change daily doesn't mean that your trainer shouldn't eventually introduce new challenges for your body. A good workout should add in some variety every 4 to 6 weeks. If added sooner, it means your trainer is guessing and doesn't have a set plan for how you can improve.

3) DO THEY KEEP GOOD RECORDS?

The best trainers learn from experience. That means every workout that has ever been performed under his or her guidance should be recorded. Your progress will be based—in part—on knowing where you started, how far you came, what worked, and what didn't. And your journey should be aided by the trainer's record of other clients who had similar situations— whether they were exercising for weight loss or training for a 5-K. If your trainer does not keep records— for you or any other client—find someone who is more organized and treats their job like a business.

4) DO THEY LOOK HOW YOU WANT TO LOOK?

It might sound superficial, but your trainer's looks do matter. Your best guarantee of results is to find a trainer who possesses a similar physique to your own, only better. That doesn't mean your trainer has to look exactly like you or even have the same body parts. But a bodybuilder is a bodybuilder and will likely train you like you're one.

5) DO THEY CONTINUE THEIR EDUCATION?

Remember that the personal training industry is a relatively young field. And between new research and the lessons learned on the training floor, conventional wisdom can change on a yearly basis. The best trainers are the ones who are constantly learning by continuing their education. Fitness seminar attendance is one of the best ways to determine whether your trainer is staying updated on how to keep you looking good and feeling healthy. Ask any potential trainer about the last seminar he or she attended. If it's been longer than three months, consider that a red flag.

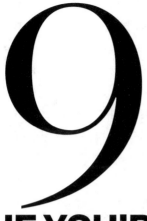

IF YOU'RE NOT HAVING FUN, YOU'RE DOING SOMETHING WRONG

HOW TO ADAPT THE *MEN'S HEALTH* MUSCLE SYSTEM TO YOUR OWN NEEDS AND MAKE SURE YOU NEVER, EVER GET SORE, TIRED, OR BORED!

The two of you used to be a perfect team. Together, you had fun. You challenged each other, and day by day you could feel yourself growing stronger and healthier and maybe even a bit wiser, too. It felt as though you had finally found the long-term relationship that would bring you eternal bliss.

But as time passed, something changed. Once, your partner inspired an unbridled bodily drive that brought you to new peaks of physical exultation. Now, you have to drag yourself to visit, and when you arrive, you just don't feel the same call, the same desire. You look in your partner's direction and all you can see is 135 pounds of dull, dead weight.

Well, don't worry. After a couple of years together, a lot of guys feel that way about their exercise equipment.

There are a lot of reasons why any great exercise partnership—with a gym, with a weight set, with a treadmill—can eventually go south. And these roadblocks to fitness affect the vast majority of us: 79 percent of men exercise less than two times week, according to the *Journal of Strength and Conditioning Research*. But the three most common reasons men cite for kicking their programs to the curb?

> **HOT TIP #97**
>
> **Go loco for coco.**
> Instead of a traditional sports drink, grab a coconut water for a post-workout boost. It's lower in calories and has loads of electrolytes and potassium.

• **LACK OF PROGRESS.** Too much work for too little reward. Lack of progress is cited in studies a lot, and there's a reason: because there are a lot of seat-of-the-pants, one-size-fits-all fitness programs out there, most of which don't take nutrition into account. (And nutrition is the bullet in any fitness plan's chamber.) Fortunately, the *Men's Health* Muscle System is a proven formula with proven results, created by our *Men's Health* fitness experts and tested by people just like you. And it wasn't until we had the eating and exercising formula just rightthat we unleashed the information in this book.

• **LACK OF TIME.** You are not idly rich. You don't have endless stretches of time to spend at the gym doing every exercise. You have a job, friends, family, and a transmission that needs to be attended to . . . about 6 months ago. You don't have time to be at the gym all day. So you need a program that is efficient, a program that will make you work hard, a program that will have you seeing results, and most of all, a program that's going to be fun. Some of these are built in to the *Men's Health* Muscle System. You'll drop the act of counting reps and be moving faster than ever—and that includes dropping fat like you never have before.

• **LACK OF EXCITEMENT.** This one's the biggie. Boredom is the balloon mortgage in your housing bubble, the intern scandal in your presidential campaign, the cracked blowout preventer in your deepwater drilling system. Unless you account for it and create a strategy plan to avoid it, it will destroy all of your best-laid plans. And here's the real bummer: The more you need to get in shape, the harder boredom fights to drag you down. No kidding: Researchers reported in the *Journal of Nutrition Education and Behavior* that people who are out of shape have a more difficult time enjoying exercise and maintaining a positive attitude about losing weight. That causes frustration, which too often leads them to quit the very thing they need most.

The other problem with boredom is that even if you manage to fight back, to stick with your same old routine, you'll eventually find that your fitness plan stops working as well as it used to. That's right, boredom actually erodes exercise gains, even if you show up for every session! In fact, scientists have found that if you stick with only one type of exercise for too long, it can decrease calorie burning by up to 25 percent. It's not that the exercises you're doing stop working; it's that you simply become bored with the same old schtick, so you work out with less intensity and don't see any changes.

So what's a red-blooded, easily bored guy supposed to do?

Brother, you came to the right place.

The Workout That Never Leaves You Bored

The basic *Men's Health* Muscle System outlined in the previous chapter is unlike any other fitness plan you've ever tried, and it's nearly—nearly—boredom proof. By getting rid of snooze-inducing exercise clichés like doing a preset number of reps and hanging around between sets, you'll be moving your body—and seeing your body change—faster than ever. And, just in case you like as much variety in your gym as Tommy Lee likes in his hotel room, this chapter includes a complete set of alternate exercises that you can swap in wherever, whenever.

But still, even the most intense, effective, revolutionary workout routine in the world is, in the end, a routine. And that's why the best way to stick to, and supercharge, your workout is to stop thinking that exercise has to involve, well, working out.

See, everything you do that involves a little bit of effort, a little bit of movement, and a little bit of fun can and should be considered exercise. So the sooner you start seeing "having fun" as an essential aspect of "exercising," the sooner you'll begin to burn fat and build muscle more effectively. In fact, a study in the journal *Sports Medicine* found that adding a wide range of activities of varying difficulty—including types of exercise that you enjoy—helps decrease boredom and increase the enjoyment of exercising. And when you enjoy exercise more, you're more likely to stick with your plan and reach your goals.

And I'm not talking just about intense, physically challenging adventures like climbing a cliff face and surfing a tsunami. Baylor University scientists found that when you combine different forms of exercise, such as mixing high- and low-intensity activity, you experience faster improvements in strength and weight loss than you would if you went balls-out every time. That means that doing a high-intensity *Men's Health* Muscle System workout one day and then a relaxing walk in the woods the next day will add just as much to your overall fitness as taking up an ax and chopping down said woods. Whether it's putting together a new grill in your backyard (20 minutes of work that will burn more than 120 calories) or running around with your kids for 15 minutes (that's another 120 calories), you'll find that engaging in your favorite everyday activities is the best way to eliminate the boredom of exercise—and change the way you look.

Your Weekly Workout Plan

Here's what you need to remember about the *Men's Health* Muscle System—you should only be lifting weights 3 days a week. And each of those workouts should take 45 minutes or less. But a good workout doesn't end when you put down the weights. In fact, that's when the fat-burning and muscle-gaining process kicks into high gear.

Don't forget, after you lift weights, your metabolism stays elevated for up to another 48 hours, and the microtears in your muscles are being repaired and growing stronger. That's why after you exercise hard, your muscles feel tight and sore. You can't extend your arms, laughing hurts your abs, and your legs feel like they were dipped in concrete. This phenomenon is called "delayed onset muscle soreness." Normally when you're feeling a bit sore, your instinct might be to cut down on your physical activity for a day or two. Besides, you worked hard at the gym—you deserve to take it easy, right?

But restricting movement is actually the worst thing for your body. It might make sense to take a day off, but the *International*

Journal of Sports Medicine found that doing low-intensity activity on your "off days" is the best way to improve recovery and increase lean muscle mass.

This is where having fun on your off day has extra benefits. Your favorite hobby helps the healing process by speeding up the flow of nutrients to your muscles, which repairs your muscle tissue. That's why it's called "active recovery," or "active rest," because it soothes your aches and pains and prepares your body for the best possible workout every time you lift weights. Another study, in the *International Journal of Sports Medicine,* found that using active recovery strategies helped cyclists perform better in subsequent training sessions than those who took a day off and performed no activity. What's more, according to a study in *Medicine and Science in Sports and Exercise*, active recovery strategies also help keep your metabolism chugging along for even more sustained fat burning. While the physical benefits are undeniable, active recovery also is essential to the mental aspect of making exercise enjoyable. A study in the *British Journal of Sports Medicine* found that low-intensity exercise on off days had a positive effect on psychological recovery by removing the monotony of traditional exercise programs and helping increase relaxation.

Each week you should make these additional activities a built-in part of your workout, in addition to your weight training. They can be things you already love to do or an activity you've never tried before. Just don't go above 60 to 70 percent of your maximum heart rate, according to researchers, and don't think that you need an all-day excursion to get the benefits: You'll be fine even with 30 minutes or so. You'll quickly find that not only will you have more energy and feel younger, but you'll also be psychologically refreshed and more excited about exercise. This will help you stay consistent and reach your goals.

DAY 1: *Men's Health* Muscle System

DAY 2: Active recovery: 20 minutes

DAY 3: *Men's Health* Muscle System

DAY 4: Day off

DAY 5: *Men's Health* Muscle System

DAY 6: Active recovery: 20 minutes

DAY 7: Day off

So what counts as an active recovery day? It can be almost any movement that gets your blood flowing. That might mean playing hoops, sweeping the floor, or wrestling with your children. The intensity can vary, but as long as you're not straining your muscles with added resistance (as you do in the *Men's Health* Muscle System), your body will benefit.

ACTIVITIES THAT COUNT AS EXERCISE ON YOUR ACTIVE RECOVERY DAY

SPORTS		HOME MAINTENANCE	HOME LIFE
BADMINTON	KAYAKING	CARPENTRY	CLEANING
BASKETBALL	ROCK CLIMBING	CAULKING	MOVING FURNITURE
BICYCLING	ROLLERBLADING/ SKATING	CLEANING RAIN GUTTERS	PLAYING WITH YOUR KIDS
BILLIARDS	RUNNING	DIGGING	
BOXING	SKIING	GARDENING	SEX (IT DOESN'T COUNT IF YOU'RE ALONE, DUDE)
DANCING	SOCCER	LAYING TILE	
FOOTBALL	SOFTBALL OR BASEBALL	MOWING LAWN	VACUUMING
FRISBEE		PAINTING	
GOLF	SWIMMING	RAKING	
HANDBALL	VOLLEYBALL	SHOVELING	
HIKING	WALKING	SWEEPING	
HORSEBACK RIDING	WATERSKIING		
JUMPING ROPE	YOGA		

So, does all this mean you can go golfing, ride a Jet Ski, play ball, try Pilates, learn to juggle, hike the Appalachian Trail, take up archery, mountain bike a back road, or wrestle an alligator only on "active recovery" days? No. As long as you give yourself at least one day of pure rest, you can do all of these fun things every day if you'd like. But the prescription here is that you need to do them at least twice a week to keep your muscles growing, your metabolism revving, and the great specter of boredom at bay.

Deal? Okay, let's go have some fun!

THREE STEPS TO
THE FASTEST RESULTS

Make your time and effort pay off—big!

1. Perform the *Men's Health* Muscle System 3 times per week.

2. Add 2 or 3 active recovery days per week, consisting of at least 20 minutes of enjoyable activity.

3. Always have at least 1 off day when you completely relax. If you feel worn out, you can to bump that up to 2 off days. Pushing your body too hard will slow you down and limit your results.

100 WAYS TO BURN 100 CALORIES

Use the guide below to learn how simple it can be to burn more calories and put yourself on the fast track to seeing your abs.

LESS THAN 5 MINUTES

- Chop wood continuously for 4 minutes, 22 seconds.
- Run a 5-minute mile. (You'll have burned 100 by 4 minutes, 30 seconds.)
- Jump on a stationary bike and ride it at a pace of 20 mph for 4 minutes, 52 seconds.

LESS THAN 10 MINUTES

- Hum the theme song to Rocky as you skip rope for 9 minutes, 30 seconds.
- Hike the great outdoors with at least 22 pounds in your backpack for 9 minutes, 15 seconds.
- Play racquetball for 7 minutes, 17 seconds.
- Swim a few laps using your favorite stroke (back, breast, or butterfly) for 8 minutes or less, depending on the stroke.
- Travel underwater instead of on top of it to burn calories even faster: Scuba dive for 7 minutes, 11 seconds.
- Hit a few on the tennis court: Play for 9 minutes.

LESS THAN 15 MINUTES

- Ski down an advanced slope.
- Tread water for 14 minutes, 30 seconds.
- Snorkel in a pool, and kick at a moderate pace (14 minutes, 5 seconds).
- Use a stationary rower for 11 minutes.
- Hit the weights for 13 minutes.
- Take an intense aerobics class and enjoy the scenery for 11 minutes, 8 seconds.
- Walk uphill for 13 minutes.

PLAYING PROFESSIONAL SPORTS

- Face LeBron James on the court for 9 minutes.
- Go two rounds with Georges St. Pierre. (Don't think you could survive that long? No problem. Lying unconscious for 1½ hours will also burn the same amount.)

- Carry Phil Mickelson's bags for two holes.
- Throw fastballs to the Chicago Cubs for two innings (14 minutes on the mound).
- Play half a period of professional hockey. (Lose calories and teeth at the same time!)
- Bowl 10 frames. (You may not bowl 300, but you'll burn 100.)
- Throw long passes while avoiding the Pittsburgh Steelers' defense for 10 minutes.
- Shoot foul shots: 207 shots at 12 shots per minute = 100 calories.

DURING A ROMANTIC EVENING

- Woo her with a 33-minute melody on the piano.
- Slow dance through seven songs (about 26 minutes).
- Give her a full-body massage for 19 minutes, 30 seconds.
- Shower her with 9,240 mini-kisses all over her body.
- Sweep her off her feet and carry her up to the bedroom. (This only works if your bedroom's on the 13th floor. If not, you burn 8 calories per flight of stairs, so walk her around a bit.)
- Make love for about an hour. (Then again, if you can accomplish this on a regular basis, chances are she doesn't care how fat you are.)
- Make breakfast in bed for her the next morning. (Includes cooking for 20 minutes, serving it to her, and, yes, doing the dishes.)

WITHOUT MOVING A MUSCLE

- Stand in line for U2 tickets for 65 minutes.
- Watch 2½ back-to-back episodes of *Seinfeld* reruns (four episodes if you have them on DVD).
- Get stuck in traffic for almost an hour.
- Sip ice water all day long. Eight 16-ounce glasses of ice water raises your metabolism (the rate at which your body burns calories) and burns an extra 100 calories.

WORKING AROUND YOUR HOUSE

- Paint the house or clean the gutters for 16 minutes.
- Rake leaves for 20 minutes.
- Push mow the lawn for 14 minutes.
- Wash and wax the station wagon for about 18 minutes.
- Shovel snow for 12 minutes, or use the snowblower for 17 minutes.
- Stack firewood for 15 minutes.
- Move boxes to the attic for 10 minutes.
- Putter around the garden for a little more than 17 minutes.

SPENDING TIME WITH THE BOYS

- Play power pool. (You'll need to shoot 10 racks at an average of 3 minutes a game.)
- Shoot some darts—four games of countdown 301 or one game of cricket.

- Play 13 hands of poker.
- Restore your buddy's classic T-Bird for 18 minutes.

AT YOUR DESK JOB

- Push a pencil for 45 minutes.
- Walk back and forth to the copier for 26 minutes.
- Type on your computer for 48 minutes.
- Talk up a client for 52 minutes.

DOING THE THINGS YOUR WIFE TELLS YOU TO DO

- Spend 13 minutes finding just the right spot for the #@*&% couch.
- Take Rex out for a 23-minute walk.
- Haul out the trash eight times.
- Lift and lower the toilet seat 3,740 times. (Just be sure to leave it down on the last one.)

DOING THE THINGS MOM TOLD YOU NOT TO DO

- Run with scissors for 9 minutes, 30 seconds.
- Talk with your mouth full for more than 38 minutes.
- Jump up and down on the bed 1,336 times.
- Wrestle with your kid brother on the living room floor for 7 minutes.

DOING THE SAME THING OVER AND OVER

- Do 97 pushups (at 10 pushups a minute).
- Do 146 crunches (at 15 crunches a minute).
- Play the nickel slots in Reno 234 times (or $11.70 worth).
- Putt 156 golf balls (at 6 putts a minute).

ACTING OUT SCENES FROM YOUR FAVORITE FILMS

- Grab a golf club and make like a swashbuckling Errol Flynn. You'll burn 100 big ones in just 8 minutes, 30 seconds (and probably break every lamp in the house).
- Groove like Travolta during a dance contest scene (Disco John in *Saturday Night Fever*: 14 minutes; '90s John in *Pulp Fiction*: 18 minutes).
- Hit the open road like Peter Fonda in *Easy Rider*: for 32 minutes.
- Reenact the climax of any martial arts movie: roughly 8 minutes.
- Defend America's pride during the Olympic table tennis scene in *Forrest Gump*: for roughly 10 minutes.
- Stand in front of the mirror and repeat "You talkin' to me? You talkin' to me?" 519 times.

GETTING IN THE CHRISTMAS SPIRIT

- Chop down five Christmas trees. (You could have a tree in every room of the house, or be generous and volunteer to do the honors for your friends and extended family.)
- Spend half an hour putting up lights outside the house.
- Roast chestnuts on an open fire (31 minutes).
- Help the kids build a snowman for 26 minutes.
- Save your Christmas shopping for the last minute: Walking briskly through a mall with a stack of packages will burn through 100 calories in just more than 19 minutes.
- Wrap 21 of those gifts when you get home.

BEING POLITICALLY CORRECT

- Plant two medium-size trees.
- Ride your bike to work (21 minutes at a leisurely pace).
- March in a protest of your choice for 10 minutes. (Carrying a sign or placard will burn even more calories.)
- Crush 623 cans for recycling.
- Volunteer to pick up trash along the highway for 19 minutes, 30 seconds.

LIVING THE GOOD LIFE

- Man a sailboat for 26 minutes.
- Wade in a heavy current while fishing for more than 12 minutes. (Don't worry if you're no good at fishing; rescuing your line from a tree is good for a quick 100 every 16 minutes.)
- Fly your private plane for 38 minutes 30 seconds.
- Read the financial section for an hour.
- Stack $560,000 worth of $100 bills into 56 piles of $10,000 each.

BEING A GOOD FATHER

- Pretend to be the bogeyman and chase a kid around for 16 minutes.
- Push your child in a stroller for 30 minutes.
- Play dodgeball or hopscotch with your children for about 15 minutes.
- Change 52 diapers.
- Dress up as Barney and greet birthday party guests for 20 minutes.
- Iron 7 shirts.
- Ice-skate with the family for 12 minutes.
- Tap your foot 9,351 times.

Three Ways to Customize the *Men's Health* Muscle System

We all hit plateaus in life. Whether you're waiting for a salary raise or trying to restart the pilot light on your relationship, exercise is no different. Sometimes you just seem to be stuck. But it doesn't have to be that way. The exercises in the *Men's Health* Muscle System were carefully selected by our top fitness advisors to maximize results in the shortest possible time. But the workout is also flexible and was created to help you achieve a better body for the rest of your life. Use the following adjustments to provide a new spin to the *Men's Health* Muscle System, so your workout never goes stale and you continually see improvements in your body.

1: Supercharge Your Metabolism

Ready to kick up your fitness another notch? Increase the difficulty of the *Men's Health* Muscle System by performing each exercise for 60 seconds (instead of 30). You'll experience more benefits with this state-of-the-art fitness system and take your body to the next level.

2: Pack on Slabs of Muscle

If you don't care about adding a few more dumbbells to your workout, you can perform each exercise for the 30-second time period using the heaviest weight you can for each exercise. So, rather than just using one pair of dumbbells for the entire workout, you will vary the weight for each exercise to build maximum strength and muscle on each lift by using dumbbells of other weights. For each exercise select a weight you could normally use for 8 to 10 repetitions.

3: Exercise Switch and Swap

The exercises in the *Men's Health* Muscle System work all of your main muscle groups from every angle while incorporating real-life movements into your program. But your workouts aren't limited to 10 exercises. Follow the original plan for at least 6 weeks, and after that time period, select any of the alternative movements from the list below and add them to your workout. Remember, you'll still perform only 10 exercises, but this will allow for more variation. You can perform nine exercises from the original workout and just change one. Or you can change all 10.

> **HOT TIP #98**
>
> **Have sex, live longer!** A study of 1000 middle-aged men found those who had the highest frequency of orgasm had a 50 percent lower death rate than those who didn't.

By adding these new movements, you'll literally create hundreds of different workouts that will have you seeing results after just a few weeks and still making improvements after a year.

Switching an exercise is like trading in one supermodel for another (which might be a problem you'll have after you follow this program for a while). The movement patterns are similar, but the new exercises will challenge your body in slightly different ways, which will help you avoid plateaus, stretch your shirtsleeves, and have you walking around bare chested even when you're not at the beach.

STANDARD EXERCISE: Dumbbell straight-leg deadlift

THE UPGRADE: Inverted hamstring

MUSCLES IT TARGETS: Hamstrings, glutes

HOW TO DO IT: Stand on your left leg with your knee bent slightly, and raise your right leg slightly off the floor behind you. Raise your arms out to the sides, with your thumbs pointing up so your body forms a T. Without changing the bend in your left knee, bend at your hips and lower your torso until it's parallel to the floor. As you bend over, make sure your arms remain at your sides with your thumbs pointing up. Your right leg should stay in line with your body as you lower your torso. Pause, then raise your torso and lowering your right leg back to the starting position. Complete all reps, then switch legs.

STANDARD EXERCISE: Dumbbell plank and row
THE UPGRADE: Dumbbell pushup and row
MUSCLES IT TARGETS: Abs, back, biceps, shoulders, chest
HOW TO DO IT: Grab a pair of hex dumbbells with an overhand grip and set yourself in pushup position, your arms straight. Lower your body to the floor, pause, then push yourself back up. Once you're back in the starting position, row the dumbbell in your right hand to the side of your chest by pulling it upward and bending your arm. Pause, then lower the dumbbell back down, and repeat the same movement with your left arm.

BONUS TOTAL BODY EXERCISE: Dumbbell pushup and arm raise
HOW TO DO IT: Grab a pair of hex dumbbells with an overhand grip and assume a pushup position, your arms straight. Lower your body to the floor and perform a pushup. Raise back up and, keeping your core stiff, reach forward with your right arm with the dumbbell in your hand. Try to prevent your body from rotating. Hold for a few seconds, then lower back down. Repeat with your left arm.

STANDARD EXERCISE: Dumbbell front squat
THE UPGRADE: Dumbbell overhead squat
MUSCLES IT TARGETS: Quads, hamstrings, glutes, shoulders, abs
HOW TO DO IT: Stand and hold a pair of dumbbells straight above your shoulders, your arms completely straight. Set your feet slightly wider than hip-width apart and brace your core. Lower your body until your thighs are at least parallel to the floor. Your

lower back should stay naturally arched for the entire movement, and don't allow the dumbbell to fall forward as you squat. Pause, and then push back to the starting position.

STANDARD EXERCISE: Dumbbell push press
THE UPGRADE: Jump squat with overhead reach
MUSCLES IT TARGETS: Quads, hamstrings, glutes, shoulders, calves
HOW TO DO IT: Holding a dumbbell in each hand, place your hands at your sides, palms facing inward, and push your hips back, bend your knees, and lower your body until your upper thighs are parallel to the floor. Pause, and then jump as high as you can. As you jump into the air, press your hands above your head as far as you can so that your arms are fully extended. Land, and then immediately squat down and repeat.

STANDARD EXERCISE: Dumbbell high pull
THE UPGRADE: Dumbbell jump shrug
MUSCLES IT TARGETS: Quads, hamstrings, glutes, shoulders, trapezius, calves
HOW TO DO IT: Grab a pair of dumbbells and let them hang at arm's length, your palms facing your sides. Bend at your hips and knees until the dumbbells hang just below your knees. Simultaneously thrust your hips forward, shrug your shoulders forcefully, and jump as high as you can. Land as softly you can, reset, and repeat.

STANDARD EXERCISE: Cross-body mountain climber
THE UPGRADE: Mountain climber
MUSCLES IT TARGETS: Abs, obliques
HOW TO DO IT: Assume a pushup position with your arms completely straight. Lift your right foot off the floor and slowly raise your knee as close to the right side of your chest as you can. Touch the floor with your right foot. Return to the starting position.

Repeat with your left leg. Alternate back and forth for the selected time period.

BONUS ABS UPGRADE: Bird dog and rotate

HOW TO DO IT: Get down on all fours and place your right hand behind your head. Extend your left leg straight out behind you. Bring your right elbow and left knee under your body so that they touch. Extend them both back to the starting position; as you do, look over your right shoulder and try to see your leg kicking behind you. Repeat on the other side. Focus on maintaining a strong core and strong glutes to keep your entire body stable.

STANDARD EXERCISE: Alternating split jump

THE UPGRADE: Dumbbell lunge

MUSCLES IT TARGETS: Quads, glutes, hamstrings

HOW TO DO IT: Grab a pair of dumbbells and hold them at your sides, your arms straight and your palms facing each other. Step forward with your left leg and slowly lower your body until your front knee is bent at least 90 degrees. Pause, then push yourself back to the starting position as quickly as you can. Repeat with your right leg.

STANDARD EXERCISE: T-pushup

THE UPGRADE: Alternating side plank

MUSCLES IT TARGETS: Abs, obliques

HOW TO DO IT: Lie on your left side with your knees straight. Prop your upper body up on your left forearm. Brace your core by contracting your abs forcefully, as if you were about to be punched in the gut. Raise your hips until your body forms a straight line from your ankles to your shoulders. This is a side plank. Hold for a moment, then rotate your body so you're in a front plank, with all of your weight on both of your elbows and your body forming a straight line from your shoulders to your ankles. Hold for another moment, then rotate onto your right forearm and perform another side plank. Keep rotating through all three planks until time is up. (Shoot for a full 2 minutes.)

BONUS CORE UPGRADE: T-rotation (without the pushup)
HOW TO DO IT: Grab a pair of hex dumbbells and assume a pushup position, your arms straight. Lift your right hand and rotate the right side of your body as you raise the dumbbell straight up over your shoulder until your body forms a T. Reverse the move and repeat, this time rotating your left side.

STANDARD EXERCISE: Reverse lunge and swing
THE UPGRADE: Dumbbell reverse lunge and rotational press.
MUSCLES IT TARGETS: Quads, glutes, hamstrings, obliques, shoulders
HOW TO DO IT: Grab a dumbbell with your left hand and hold it next to your left shoulder, your palm facing in. Step backward with your left leg and lower your body into a reverse lunge as you simultaneously press the dumbbell straight above your left shoulder. As you press the dumbbell overhead, rotate your torso to the right. Return to the start, hold the dumbbell in your right hand, and repeat.

STANDARD EXERCISE: Dumbbell row
THE UPGRADE: Alternating dumbbell row
MUSCLES IT TARGETS: Back, biceps
HOW TO DO IT: Grab a pair of dumbbells, bend at your hips and knees, and lower your torso until it's almost parallel to the floor. Let the dumbbells hang at arm's length from your shoulders, your palms facing you. Instead of rowing both dumbbells up at once, lift them one at a time, in an alternating fashion. As you lift one dumbbell, lower the other, without allowing your back to round.

Boredom can erode exercise gains and decrease calorie burning by up to 25 percent.

10

THE 250 BEST FOODS FOR MEN
THE ULTIMATE GUIDE TO EATING THE VERY BEST, NO MATTER WHERE YOU ARE OR WHAT YOU HANKER FOR!

You will never own the world's biggest yacht. (That would be the 557-foot Eclipse, owned by Russian billionaire Roman Abramovich.)

You will never live on the top floor of the world's tallest skyscraper. (It's the 2,717-foot-tall Burj Khalifa in Dubai, with its 4,000 tons of steel.)

You will never share your life with the world's most desirable woman. (Brad Pitt, Jay-Z, and Tom Brady appear to be battling it out for that honor.)

But when it comes to having the absolute best—no compromises, no excuses, no competition—there's one place where you can score just as big as the Arab princes, the rap moguls, the movie stars, and the sports wizards.

You can—you will—eat the very best food in the world.

Those guys might have legions of assistants, armies of accountants, even harems of women to help them meet their goals. But you have one thing they don't have: You have the editors of *Men's Health* on your side.

For more than 20 years, we've been analyzing, calculating, investigating, and assembling a list of the very best foods in the world. From the finest fast-food fries to the ultimate instant oatmeal to the perfect penne pasta, we've tested and tasted it and listed it here for you. And, as publishers of the *Eat This, Not That!* series of nutrition guides, we have access to the largest database of commercial foods ever assembled.

A lot of factors went into creating this ultimate list. And while calories were a big part of our calculations, we refused to compromise on taste or nutritional content—a few extra grams of protein or fiber are usually worth a few dozen calories, especially in the nutritionally sparse landscape of American restaurants.

As you'll remember from Chapter 6, expanding the *Men's Health* Nutrition System to include the perfect antidote to any craving—the most nutritious food, the best-tasting food—is one of the hallmarks of *The Men's Health Diet*, a crucial Rule of the Ripped that will guarantee you live fitter, leaner, longer.

Striving for the best at all times ought to be your goal. Every time you choose something that's less than the best, remember: Jay-Z, Brad Pitt, and a Russian billionaire are all laughing at you....

The Very Best Foods At The Supermarket

BREADS AND GRAINS

1. Best Cereal
Kashi Whole-Wheat Biscuits, Cinnamon Harvest
One bowl contains all the fiber you need to stay full until lunch.
PER 2 OZ (28 BISCUITS): 180 calories, 6 g protein, 43 g carbs (5 g fiber, 9 g sugars), 1 g fat, 0 g sodium

2. Best Instant Oatmeal
Quaker Weight Control Instant Oatmeal, Cinnamon
This morning meal has a sane number of calories and won't jolt your taste buds with too much sugar.
PER PACKET: 160 calories, 7 g protein, 29 g carbs (6 g fiber, 1 g sugars), 3 g fat, 290 mg sodium

3. Best Steel-Cut Oats
Arrowhead Mills Organic Steel Cut Oats Hot Cereal
It's nuttier and more filling than instant oatmeal.
PER ¼ CUP: 160 calories, 6 g protein, 27 g carbs (8 g fiber, 0 g sugars), 3 g fat, 0 mg sodium

4. Best Granola
Nature's Path Organic Pomegran Plus Granola with Cherries
Mix into Greek yogurt (# 31) for an easy postworkout snack.
PER ¾ CUP: 250 calories, 5 g protein, 38 g carbs (4 g fiber, 13 g sugars), 9 g fat, 60 mg sodium

5. Best Breakfast Bar
KIND Plus Almond Cashew + Flax (Omega-3)
A crunchy, craving-busting bar with just nine ingredients—all of which you can pronounce.
PER BAR: 150 calories, 4 g protein, 18 g carbs (4 g fiber, 14 g sugars), 9 g fat, 0 mg sodium

6. Best Bagel
Pepperidge Farm Whole Grain
Include a scrambled egg with one of these for a protein-packed start to your day.
PER BAGEL: 250 calories, 11 g protein, 49 g carbs (6 g fiber, 9 g sugars), 1.5 g fat, 450 mg sodium

7. Best English Muffin
Rudi's Organic Whole Grain Wheat English Muffins
Upgrade your breakfast: Top it with tomato, egg, and a slice of Swiss (#23).
PER MUFFIN: 120 calories, 5 g protein, 23 g carbs (3 g fiber, 2 g sugars), 1 g fat, 220 mg sodium

8. Best Sliced Bread
Arnold Grains & More Bread, 100% Whole Wheat Triple Health
No high-fructose corn syrup and plenty of fiber.
PER SLICE: 100 calories, 4 g protein, 20 g carbs (6 g fiber, 3 g sugars), 2 g fat, 170 mg sodium

9. Best Burger Bun
Arnold Select Sandwich Thins,
Whole Wheat
*Don't let the bread overwhelm your
sandwich. These thin buns save on
calories so you can layer on protein.*
PER BUN: 100 calories, 5 g protein,
21 g carbs (5 g fiber, 2 g sugars),
1 g fat, 230 mg sodium

10. Best Hot Dog Roll
Pepperidge Farm Classic
Whole Grain White
*A tasty bun that stands up to what-
ever you top your dog with.*
PER ROLL: 110 calories, 6 g protein,
21 g carbs (2 g fiber, 2 g sugars),
1 g fat, 220 mg sodium

11. Best Tortilla
La Tortilla Factory Smart &
Delicious Extra Virgin Olive Oil
Multi–Grain Soft Wrap
*Wrap slices of avocado, lettuce,
tomato, and cooked bacon (#115)
in this tortilla for an awesome
riff on a BLT.*
PER TORTILLA: 100 calories,
9 g protein, 18 g carbs (12 g fiber,
1 g sugars), 3.5 g fat, 290 mg sodium

12. Best Pita
Weight Watchers
100% Whole Wheat
Perfect for a sandwich on the go.
PER PITA: 100 calories, 7 g protein,
24 g carbs (9 g fiber, 0 g sugars),
1 g fat, 260 mg sodium

13. Best Pizza Crust
Rustic Crust Organic Great Grains
*Think outside the box: Top your pizza
with thinly sliced potatoes, chopped
leeks, prosciutto, and blue cheese
crumbles. Bake at 450°F for 15 minutes or until crispy.*
PER ⅛ CRUST: 140 calories,
5 g protein, 28 g carbs (5 g fiber, 0 g sugars),
1.5 g fat, 190 mg sodium

14. Best Whole-Wheat Pasta
Bionaturae Organic
Whole Wheat Spaghetti
*A whole-wheat pasta that doesn't
taste like the box from which it came.*
PER 2 OZ: 180 calories, 7 g protein,
35 g carbs (6 g fiber, 1 g sugars),
1.5 g fat, 0 mg sodium

15. Best Regular Pasta
Ronzoni Smart Taste
Thin Spaghetti
*It's smart because it has as much
calcium as a glass of milk and three
times the fiber of regular pasta.*
PER 2 OZ: 180 calories, 6 g protein,
43 g carbs (7 g fiber, 1 g sugars),
0.5 g fat, 5 mg sodium

16. Best Quick-Cooking Rice
Uncle Ben's Ready
Whole Grain Brown
*The easiest side dish ever.
Microwave for 90 seconds and you're
good to go.*
PER CUP: 240 calories, 5 g protein,
39 g carbs (2 g fiber, 0 g sugars),
3 g fat, 15 mg sodium

17. Best Grain

Bob's Red Mill Organic
Whole Grain Quinoa
*Switch up your sides by swapping it
for rice.*

PER ¼ CUP: 170 calories, 7 g protein,
30 g carbs (3 g fiber, 0 g sugars),
2.5 g fat, 2 mg sodium

18. Best Flour

King Arthur Flour 100% Organic
Unbleached White Whole Wheat
*Rich in fiber just like regular
whole-wheat flour but with a lighter
flavor. Perfect for making homemade
pizza dough.*

PER ¼ CUP: 100 calories, 4 g protein,
18 g carbs (3 g fiber, <1 g sugars),
0.5 g fat, 0 mg sodium

DAIRY AND DELI

19. Best Milk

Organic Valley
Reduced Fat 2%
*A little fat in your milk may help
you absorb vitamins.*

PER CUP: 130 calories, 8 g protein,
13 g carbs (0 g fiber, 12 g sugars),
5 g fat, 125 mg sodium

20. Best Chocolate Milk

Horizon Reduced Fat 2%
*Drink this postworkout: Its combo
of carbs and protein can help repair
your muscles.*

PER CUP: 180 calories, 8 g protein,
27 g carbs (<1 fiber, 27 g sugars),
5 g fat, 160 mg sodium

21. Best All-Purpose Cheese

Bella Rosa Parmigiano Reggiano
*Grate this sharp Italian cheese
on everything from pasta to pizza
to soup.*

PER GRATED TBSP: 20 calories,
2 g protein, N/A carbs, 1.5 g fat, N/A sodium

22. Best High-End Cheese

Emmi Le Gruyere
Cave-Aged Kaltbach
*Pair this rich and luscious cheese
(available in many supermarkets)
with an apple for the ultimate snack.*

PER OZ: 120 calories, 8 g protein,
0 g carbs, 9 g fat, 160 mg sodium

23. Best Sandwich Cheese

Jarlsberg Lite Reduced Fat
Swiss Cheese, Deli Fresh Slices
*Well-rounded flavor without the
high sodium content of processed
American cheese.*

PER SLICE: 50 calories, 7 g protein,
0 g carbs, 2.5 g fat, 100 mg sodium

24. Best Shredded Cheese

Organic Valley Reduced Fat
Monterey Jack Cheese
*It tastes great and melts well, unlike
other low-fat cheeses.*

PER ¼ CUP: 80 calories, 8 g protein,
1 g carbs (0 g fiber, 0 g sugars),
5 g fat, 180 mg sodium

25. Best Snacking Cheese

Laughing Cow Mini Babybel, Light
*Keep a few in your work tote
(in an insulated container) to fight
on-the-job hunger.*

PER PIECE: 50 calories, 6 g protein,
0 g carbs, 3 g fat, 160 mg sodium

26. **Best Cream Cheese**
Philadelphia Whipped
Cream Cheese
*With a third fewer calories than
regular Philadelphia cream cheese—
and all the flavor—you can schmear
without fear.*
PER 2 TBSP: 60 calories, 1 g protein,
1 g carbs (0 g fiber, <1 g sugars),
6 g fat, 90 mg sodium

27. **Best Cottage Cheese**
Friendship Lowfat Cottage Cheese
*Our tasters noted this brand has
more curds and less liquid than
others, for a more satisfying snack.*
PER ½ CUP: 90 calories, 16 g protein,
3 g carbs (0 g fiber, 3 g sugars),
1 g fat, 360 mg sodium

28. **Best Sour Cream**
Breakstone's All Natural
*Stir in the juice and zest of a lime
and some chopped scallions to make
an awesome taco topping.*
PER 2 TBSP: 60 calories, 1 g protein,
1 g carbs (0 g fiber, 1 g sugars),
5 g fat, 10 mg sodium

29. **Best Butter**
Keller's Whipped Butter, Salted
*Big butter flavor, with more air
(hence fewer calories) than your
typical stick of butter.*
PER TBSP: 70 calories, 0 g protein,
0 g carbs, 7 g fat, 55 mg sodium

30. **Best Butter Spread**
Keller's Spreadable Butter
with Canola Oil
*Our tasters agree: This brand
tastes like the real deal, and spreads
easily.*
PER TBSP: 100 calories, 0 g protein,
0 g carbs, 11 g fat, 80 mg sodium

31. **Best Plain Yogurt**
Stonyfield Farm Oikos Organic
Greek Yogurt, Plain
*Throw in some blueberries, and
add a drizzle of honey if you like your
yogurt sweet.*
PER 5.3-OZ CONTAINER: 80 calories,
15 g protein, 6 g carbs (0 g fiber,
6 g sugars), 0 g fat, 60 mg sodium

32. **Best Flavored Yogurt**
Chobani Nonfat Strawberry
Greek Yogurt
*Thick, creamy, and sweet. Think
of it as a healthy dessert.*
PER 6-OZ CONTAINER: 140 calories,
14 g protein, 20 g carbs (1 g fiber,
19 g sugars), 0 g fat, 65 mg sodium

33. **Best Probiotic Yogurt**
Lifeway Lowfat Raspberry Kefir
*This fruity, drinkable probiotic
didn't have a gross aftertaste like
some of the others we tried.*
PER CUP: 160 calories, 11 g protein,
25 g carbs (3 g fiber, 21 g sugars),
125 mg sodium

34. Best Eggs

Eggland's Best Organic

Fry one up for your morning toast: The rich yellow yolk packs great flavor.

PER LARGE EGG: 70 calories, 6 g protein, 0 g carbs, 4 g fat, 60 mg sodium

35. Best Cold Cuts

Applegate Farms Organic Roasted Turkey Breast

Juicy, flavorful deli turkey.

PER 2 OZ: 50 calories, 10 g protein, 1 g carbs (0 g fiber, 0 g sugars), 360 mg sodium

36. Best Pepperoni

Hormel Turkey 70% Less Fat

Perfect as an out-of-the-bag snack. More satisfying than potato chips, too.

PER 17 SLICES: 70 calories, 9 g protein, 0 g carbs, 4 g fat, 640 mg sodium

FROZEN FOODS

37. Best Frozen Appetizer

Annie Chun's Chicken & Garlic Mini Wontons

They're easier on your belly than mozzarella sticks.

PER 4 WONTONS: 60 calories, 3 g protein, 9 g carbs (1 g fiber, 1 g sugars), 0.5 g fat, 150 mg sodium

38. Best Beef Entrée

Stouffer's Beef Pot Roast

One of the few selections that tastes like beef. A little high on sodium, so watch your portions.

PER PACKAGE: 320 calories, 20 g protein, 41 g carbs (8 g fiber, 9 g sugars), 8 g fat, 1,570 mg sodium

39. Best Chicken Entrée

Kashi Red Curry Chicken

Miraculously, this Thai-inspired dish doesn't taste like a frozen meal, and the combo of sweet potato, bok choy, and kale adds flavor as well as fiber.

PER PACKAGE: 300 calories, 18 g protein, 40 g carbs (5 g fiber, 10 g sugars), 9 g fat, 470 mg sodium

40. Best Fish Entrée

Seapak Roasted Garlic Encrusted Flounder

For a great fish sandwich, pair with mayo (#74), lemon, and cilantro

PER FILLET: 300 calories, 19 g protein, 40 g carbs (1 g fiber, 14 g sugars), 7 g fat, 1,010 mg sodium

41. Best Pasta Entrée

Kashi Pesto Pasta Primavera

A good mix of whole-grain pasta, basil pesto, and an assortment of vegetables.

PER MEAL: 290 calories, 11 g protein, 37 g carbs (7 g fiber, 4 g sugars), 11 g fat, 750 mg sodium

42. Best Vegetarian Entrée

Amy's Black Bean Enchilada Dinner

Meatless protein from beans, corn, rice, and tofu combine for a satisfying Mexican meal that's way healthier than the typical burrito.

PER PACKAGE: 330 calories, 9 g protein, 53 g carbs (9 g fiber, 4 g sugars), 8 g fat, 740 mg sodium

43. **Best Pizza**
Amy's Cheese Pizza
Make it even tastier by adding thinly sliced onions and peppers two minutes before it's done.
PER ⅓ PIZZA: 290 calories, 12 g protein, 33 g carbs (2 g fiber, 4 g sugars), 12 g fat, 590 mg sodium

44. **Best Burrito**
Evol Burritos Cilantro Lime Chicken
Free-range chicken, organic black beans, real salsa. What's not to love?
PER BURRITO: 320 calories, 16 g protein, 49 g carbs (4 g fiber, 1 g sugars), 7 g fat, 450 mg sodium

45. **Best Vegetarian Burger**
Gardenburger GardenVegan
It's best cooked on the grill or in a skillet with a teaspoon of canola oil (#118). Top it with a few slices of fresh avocado.
PER PATTY: 80 calories, 9 g protein, 12 g carbs (4 g fiber, 0 g sugars), 1 g fat, 270 mg sodium

46. **Best Fish Sticks**
Dr. Praeger's Sensible Foods Fish Sticks, Potato Crusted
Try them sprinkled with lemon juice, freshly ground black pepper (#122), and chopped parsley for a more sophisticated meal.
PER 3 STICKS: 120 calories, 6 g protein, 7 g carbs (<1 g fiber, 0 g sugars), 8 g fat, 220 mg sodium

47. **Best French Fries**
Cascadian Farm Crinkle Cut French Fries
No partially hydrogenated oil (a.k.a. trans fat).
PER 18 PIECES: 110 calories, 2 g protein, 17 g carbs (2 g fiber, 1 g sugars), 4 g fat, 10 mg sodium

48. **Best Breakfast Sandwich**
Weight Watchers Smart Ones Morning Express Breakfast Quesadilla
A good source of protein and fiber—which means it'll keep you full until lunch.
PER QUESADILLA: 230 calories, 12 g protein, 29 g carbs (6 g fiber, 1 g sugars), 7 g fat, 730 mg sodium

49. **Best Waffle**
Van's 8 Whole Grains Multigrain
Top these fiber-rich waffles with yogurt (#31) and fruit for a satisfying breakfast.
PER 2 WAFFLES: 180 calories, 3 g protein, 31 g carbs (6 g fiber, 3 g sugars), 7 g fat, 320 mg sodium

50. **Best Vegetable**
Cascadian Farm Organic Garden Peas
You don't even need butter—these peas require only a pinch of sea salt (#121) to taste amazing.
PER ⅔ CUP: 70 calories, 4 g protein, 12 g carbs (4 g fiber, 4 g sugars), 0 g fat, 95 mg sodium

51. **Best Fruit**
Whole Foods 365 Everyday Value Organic Berry Blend
Keep a bag on hand for smoothies.
PER ¾ CUP: 70 calories, 1 g protein, 15 g carbs (3 g fiber, 10 g sugars), 0 g fat, 0 mg sodium

52. **Best Ice Cream**
Breyers Smooth & Dreamy All Natural ½ Fat Vanilla Bean
Skip the chunks and swirls. This ice cream has enough flavor to stand on its own.
PER ½ CUP: 110 calories, 3 g protein, 16 g carbs (0 g fiber, 16 g sugars), 3.5 g fat, 50 mg sodium

53. **Best Frozen Treat**
Edy's Fruit Bars (Variety Pack: Lime, Strawberry, Wildberry)
Real fruit trumps artificial flavor in a low-calorie pop. A great guilt-free snack.
PER BAR: 60 calories, 0 g protein, 13 g carbs (0 g fiber, 13 g sugars), 0 g fat, 0 mg sodium

JARRED AND CANNED GOODS

54. **Best Soup**
Lucini Italia Rustic Italian Minestrone Soup
Filled with chunks of hearty vegetables.
PER CUP: 160 calories, 5 g protein, 22 g carbs (4 g fiber, 6 g sugars), 7 g fat, 760 mg sodium

55. **Best Chili**
Amy's Organic Low-Fat Medium Black Bean
Plenty of fiber, with just the right amount of spice.
PER CUP: 200 calories, 13 g protein, 31 g carbs (13 g fiber, 3 g sugars), 3 g fat, 680 mg sodium

56. **Best Refried Beans**
Eden Organic Spicy Refried Black Beans
These spicy beans have more flavor than regular canned beans and, despite the "refried" part, only a bit of added fat.
PER ½ CUP: 110 calories, 6 g protein, 18 g carbs (7 g fiber, 0 g sugars), 1.5 g fat, 180 mg sodium

57. **Best Canned Beans**
Eden Organic Black Beans
Simmer these antioxidant-rich beans with sautéed onions and peppers for an easy side.
PER ½ CUP: 110 calories, 7 g protein, 18 g carbs (6 g fiber, 0 g sugars), 1 g fat, 15 mg sodium

58. **Best Canned Tomatoes**
Cento San Marzano Organic Peeled Tomatoes
Chop these tomatoes until slightly chunky for the perfect pizza sauce.
PER ½ CUP: 25 calories, 1 g protein, 5 g carbs (2 g fiber, 4 g sugars), 0 g fat, 20 mg sodium

59. **Best Olives**
Mezzetta Jalapeño Stuffed Olives
Just one, straight out of the jar, makes an instant salty-spicy snack–or a great addition to a martini. For an amazing salsa, chop some up and mix them with diced tomatoes and cilantro.
PER OLIVE: 10 calories, N/A protein, 1 g carbs (N/A fibers, N/A sugars), 1 g fat, N/A sodium

60. **Best Pickle**
Woodstock Farms Organic Kosher Whole Dill Pickles
Crispier and tastier than typical jarred varieties. Slide one of these alongside your next sandwich.
PER PICKLE: 10 calories, 0 g protein, 2 g carbs (0 g fiber, 0 g sugars), 0 g fat, 580 mg sodium

61. **Best Ready-to-Eat Tuna**
Starkist Tuna, Chunk Light in Water
A perfect match for a toasted English muffin (#7).
PER 2.6-OZ POUCH: 80 calories, 18 g protein, 1 g carbs (1 g fiber, 0 g sugars), 0.5 g fat, 300 mg sodium

62. **Best Ready-to-Eat Salmon**
Bumble Bee Premium Wild Pink Salmon
A good source of heart-healthy omega-3 fatty acids.
PER 2 OZ: 60 calories, 14 g protein, 0 g carbs, 1.5 g fat, 180 mg sodium

SPREADS, DIPS, AND TOPPINGS

63. **Best Ketchup**
Heinz Organic
This version of the classic ketchup tastes fresher and brighter than the nonorganic variety.
PER TBSP: 20 calories, 5 g carbs (0 g fiber, 4 g sugars), 0 g fat, 190 mg sodium

64. **Best Mustard**
Annie's Naturals Organic Dijon Mustard
Spread it on a sandwich instead of mayo, or make a quick homemade salad dressing: Blend ½ tablespoon of mustard and two tablespoons of lemon juice, then whisk in ¼ cup extra-virgin olive oil (#119) until smooth. Season with salt and freshly ground pepper.
PER TBSP: 5 calories, 0 g protein, 1 g carbs (N/A fiber, N/A sugars), 0 g fat, 120 mg sodium

65. **Best Mayonnaise**
Kraft with Olive Oil Reduced Fat
For a killer spicy mayo that'll wake up your sandwich, combine this with hot sauce (#117) to taste.
PER TBSP: 45 calories, 2 g carbs (0 g fiber, 1 g sugars), 4 g fat, 95 mg sodium

66. Best Barbecue Sauce

Pork Barrel

Brush this relatively low-calorie sauce on chicken just minutes before it comes off the grill for a tangy, smoky flavor, or drizzle it over a roast-pork sandwich.

PER 2 TBSP: 35 calories, <1 g protein, 8 g carbs (0 g fiber, 7 g sugars), 390 mg sodium

67. Best Steak Sauce

Peter Luger Steak House Old Fashioned Sauce

Upgrade your steak with the tangy, lightly spicy sauce from Brooklyn's iconic chophouse.

PER TBSP: 30 calories, 0 g protein, 7 g carbs (0 g fiber, 7 g sugars), 0 g fat, 125 mg sodium

68. Best Marinade

Wild Thymes Tropical Mango Lime

It gives fish, chicken, other meats, and vegetables a flavor kick without adding too many calories.

PER TBSP: 12 calories, <1 g protein, 3 g carbs (1 g fiber, 2 g sugars), 0 g fat, 31 mg sodium

69. Best Tomato Sauce

La Famiglia DelGrosso Pasta Sauce, Chef John's Tomato Basil Masterpiece

It tastes like fresh tomatoes; not sugary like most jarred sauces.

PER ½ CUP: 70 calories, 1 g protein, 8 g carbs (2 g fiber, 5 g sugars), 4 g fat, 300 mg sodium

70. Best Salsa

Santa Barbara Salsa (Medium)

Unlike many other jarred and fresh salsas we tested, this one was not too sweet or salty, with a fresh, chunky texture.

PER OZ: 10 calories, 0 g protein, 2 g carbs (0 g fiber, 1 g sugars), 0 g fat, 170 mg sodium

71. Best Guacamole

Yucatan Organic Guacamole

Some "guacamole flavor" dips contain little actual avocado. This brand lists organic Hass avocados as the first ingredient.

PER 2 TBSP: 60 calories, 1 g protein, 3 g carbs (2 g fiber, 1 g sugars), 4.5 g fat, 170 mg sodium

72. Best Peanut Butter

Once Again Organic American Classic Creamy

Slather on a waffle (#49) for a tasty and filling breakfast.

PER 2 TBSP: 190 calories, 7 g protein, 7 g carbs (2 g fiber, 2 g sugars), 15 g fat, 55 mg sodium

73. Best Jam/Fruit Spread

Dickinson's Organic Strawberry Fruit Spread

Spoon onto vanilla ice cream (#52) for the perfect sundae.

PER TBSP: 45 calories, 0 g protein, 11 g carbs (0 g fiber, 11 g sugars), 0 g fat, 0 mg sodium

74. **Best Condiment**

Flora Sundried Tomato Bruschetta
Brush on baguette slices and top with fresh mozzarella, prosciutto, and basil, or stir into pasta with roasted vegetables.
PER 2 TBSP: 150 calories, 7 g protein, <1 g carbs (0 g fiber, <1 g sugars), 13 g fat, 190 mg sodium

75. **Best Dip**

Summer Fresh Baba Ghanouj Creamy Roasted Eggplant Dip
This smooth Middle Eastern dip tastes great with warmed pita.
PER 2 TBSP: 110 calories, 1 g protein, 1 g carbs (0 g fiber, 0 g sugars), 12 g fat, 180 mg sodium

76. **Best Hummus**

Cedar's Original Hommus Tahini
Creamy, with a punch of garlic. Add a drizzle of olive oil (#119) to enhance the flavors.
PER 2 TBSP: 60 calories, 2 g protein, 4 g carbs (1 g fiber, 1 g sugars), 4.5 g fat, 115 mg sodium

77. **Best Salad Dressing**

Drew's Roasted Garlic & Peppercorn Salad Dressing
Unlike most creamy dressings, this one's light enough not to clobber the flavor of the rest of the salad.
PER TBSP: 70 calories, 0 g protein, 0 g carbs, 8 g fat, 69 mg sodium

78. **Best Pancake Syrup**

Spring Tree 100% Pure All Natural Maple Syrup Grade A Dark Amber
Real maple syrup doesn't have high-fructose corn syrup or a cloying aftertaste.
PER TBSP: 53 calories, 13 carbs

SNACKS

79. **Best Pretzel**

Herr's Pretzel Sticks, Whole Grain, Honey Wheat
The fiber in this snack will help fill you up.
PER 7 PRETZELS: 110 calories, 3 g protein, 22 g carbs (4 g fiber, 2 g sugars), 1 g fat, 300 mg sodium

80. **Best Tortilla Chip**

Miguel's Organic Everything Tortilla Dippers
Our tasters went back for seconds.
PER 10 CHIPS: 140 calories, 2 g protein, 18 g carbs (2 g fiber, 0 g sugars), 7 g fat, 80 mg sodium

81. **Best Potato Chip**

Pop Chips Cheddar Potato
Popped with air, not fried, for a better sandwich side.
PER 20 CHIPS: 120 calories, 2 g protein, 20 g carbs (1 g fiber, 1 g sugars), 4 g fat, 290 mg sodium

82. **Best Cracker**

Kashi Original 7 Grain Snack Crackers
Dip into hummus (#76) for a healthy mid-afternoon snack.
PER 15 CRACKERS: 120 calories, 3 g protein, 21 g carbs (2 g fiber, 3 g sugars), 3.5 g fat, 160 mg sodium

83. **Best Popcorn**

Half Naked Popcorn
(made with olive oil)
*Air-popped and dressed with just a
touch of heart-healthy olive oil, it's
the perfect movie snack.*

PER 4 CUPS: 120 calories, 3 g protein,
21 g carbs (4 g fiber, 4 g sugars),
3 g fat, 140 mg sodium

84. **Best Jerky**

Matador Beef Jerky, Original
*Pack it in your gym bag—jerky is
a delicious on-the-go fat-fighting
protein snack.*

PER OZ: 80 calories, 11 g protein,
6 g carbs (0 g fiber, 5 g sugars),
1.5 g fat, 610 mg sodium

85. **Best Nut**

Planters Nut–rition Almonds
*For an instant tummy-filling snack,
reach for these nuts, seasoned only
with sea salt.*

PER 28 G (ABOUT 2 TBSP):
170 calories, 6 g protein, 6 g carbs
(3 g fiber, 1 g sugars), 15 g fat,
40 mg sodium

86. **Best Nut Alternative**

Eden Organic Pumpkin Seeds
*A high-protein snack you can take
anywhere.*

PER ¼ CUP: 200 calories,
10 g protein, 5 g carbs (5 g fiber, 0 g sugars),
16 g fat, 100 mg sodium

87. **Best Dried Fruit**

Peeled Snacks
Much-Ado-About-Mango
*No added sugar or artificial flavors,
and only one ingredient: mango.*

PER 1.4-OZ BAG: 120 calories,
2 g protein, 28 g carbs (2 g fiber,
20 g sugars), 0 g fat, 0 mg sodium

88. **Best Trail Mix**

Sahale Snacks
Southwest Cashews
*Not your forest ranger's gorp:
This tangy mix is flavored with chili
powder and cheddar cheese.*

PER ¼ CUP: 140 calories, 5 g protein,
10 g carbs (1 g fiber, 3 g sugars),
10 g fat, 270 mg sodium

89. **Best Snack Bar**

Lärabar Peanut Butter Cookie
*The perfect way to power through
to a late lunch.*

PER BAR: 220 calories, 7 g protein,
23 g carbs (4 g fiber, 18 g sugars),
12 g fat, 45 mg sodium

90. **Best Chocolate Bar**

Dagoba's Organic Beacoup Berries
*Dried fruit boosts flavor and
antioxidants.*

PER BAR: 250 calories, 5 g protein,
27 g carbs (7 g fiber, 18 g sugars),
19 g fat, 0 mg sodium

91. **Best Cookie**

Country Choice Organic
Soft Baked Double Fudge
Brownie Cookies
*Rich and chewy—without calorie
overload.*

PER COOKIE: 90 calories, 1 g protein,
16 g carbs (1 g fiber, 10 g sugars),
3 g fat, 80 mg sodium

DRINKS

92. **Best Bottled Water**
Fiji
When you're not pouring purified water into a reusable canteen, pick up this water: Our tasters preferred its clean, crisp flavor above other brands.
0 calories

93. **Best Sports Drink**
Zico Pure Coconut Water with Mango
An 11-ounce serving packs more potassium than a banana (and a lot more than your average sports drink), all for a modest calorie count.
PER 11 OZ: 60 calories, 1 g protein, 15 g carbs (0 g fiber, 14 g sugars), 0 g fat, 60 mg sodium

94. **Best Flavored Water**
Poland Spring Sparkling Water with Lemon Essence
Kick your soda cravings for good with this carbonated water that has a hint of flavoring but no sugar.
0 calories

95. **Best Fruit Juice**
Simply Grapefruit
Naturally lower in sugar than other fruit juices and loaded with lycopene, it's the most underrated juice in the cooler. Mix it with sparkling water (#94) for a healthy riff on soda.
PER 8 OZ: 90 calories, 1 g protein, 21 g carbs (0 g fiber, 18 g sugars), 0 g fat, 10 mg sodium

96. **Best Vegetable Juice**
V8 100% Vegetable Juice, Low Sodium
This low-salt version (only 140 milligrams of sodium per cup) actually tastes better than the full-sodium version.
PER 8 OZ: 50 calories, 2 g protein, 10 carbs (2 g fiber, 8 g sugars), 0 g fat, 140 mg sodium

97. **Best Bottled Smoothie**
Bolthouse Farms Berry Boost
Not eating enough fruit? Drink this blend of blackberries, boysenberries, and raspberries.
PER 8 OZ: 130 calories, 0 g protein, 30 g carbs (4 g fiber, 21 g sugars), 1 g fat, 20 mg sodium

98. **Best Bottled Tea**
Honest Tea Organic Honey Green Tea
This tea has more metabolism-boosting, cancer-fighting catechins than its competitors.
PER 8 OZ: 35 calories, 0 g protein, 9 g carbs (0 g fiber, 9 g sugars), 5 mg sodium

99. **Best Caffeinated Bag Tea**
Numi Organic Aged Earl Grey Black Tea
This aged tea is more robust than your grandma's variety and bold enough to sub in for your morning coffee.
0 calories

100. **Best Herbal Bag Tea**
Stash Peppermint
Peppermint packs disease-fighting antioxidants and may help calm an upset stomach.
0 calories

101. Best Coffee

Illy Ground Coffee

A dark roast that brews up beautifully.

0 calories

102. Best Instant Coffee

Starbucks VIA Ready Brew

Be your own barista: Pour a packet into your mug, add hot water, and stir. No pot needed.

0 calories

103. Best Beer

Hoegaarden

A light-bodied Belgian brew with hints of spice and orange. It'll satisfy beer snobs—and regular folks, too.

PER 11.2 OZ: 176 calories, N/A protein, 13.4 g carbs (N/A fiber, N/A sugars), N/A fat, N/A sodium

104. Best Microbrew

Bell's Hopslam

This microbrewery's intense double India pale ale is flavorful and satisfyingly bitter. It deserves to be savored.

PER 12 OZ: 280 calories, N/A protein, N/A carbs (N/A fiber, N/A sugars), N/A fat, N/A sodium

105. Best Low-Calorie Beer

Guinness Draught

Dark does not equal heavy. This smooth Irish brew may have a few more calories than most light beers, but it also packs much more satisfaction.

PER 12 OZ: 126 calories, N/A protein, 10 g carbs (N/A fiber, N/A sugars), N/A fat, N/A sodium

106. Best Red Wine Under $20

Louis M. Martini Cabernet Sauvignon, Sonoma County, 2007

Delivers rich flavors of black cherry, blackberry, and fresh sage—and won't make a big dent in your paycheck.

PER 4 OZ: 98 calories, N/A protein, 4 g carbs, (N/A fiber, N/A sugars), N/A fat, N/A sodium

107. Best White Wine Under $15

Pacific Rim Dry Riesling, Columbia Valley, 2007

This versatile bargain bottle grabbed our attention with the apricot flavors that stand up even to Thai takeout.

PER 4 OZ: 86 calories, 1 g carbs

PROTEIN

108. Best Hot Dog

Applegate Farms Uncured Beef Hot Dogs

No nitrates means less chance that you'll develop a postmeal headache.

PER DOG: 80 calories, 5 g protein, 0 g carbs, 6 g fat, 380 mg sodium

109. Best Chicken

Bell & Evans Organic Boneless/ Skinless Breast Meat

The juiciest, most flavorful supermarket poultry we tasted.

PER 4 OZ: 120 calories, 27 g protein, 0 g carbs, 1.5 g fat, 70 mg sodium

110. **Best Steak**
Laura's Lean Beef
Ribeye Steak
Lean and succulent.
PER 4 OZ: 175 calories, 24 g protein,
0 g carbs, 9 g fat, 70 mg sodium

111. **Best Ground Beef**
Laura's Beef 92% Lean Ground
For great burgers, all this humanely raised meat needs is a dash of salt and pepper.
PER 4 OZ: 160 calories, 21 g protein,
0 g carbs, 9 g fat, 70 mg sodium

112. **Best Turkey**
Diestel Boneless, Skinless
Turkey, Dark Meat
Diestel's turkeys are plumped on a natural vegetarian diet.
PER 4 OZ: 130 calories, 23 g protein,
0 g carbs, 3 g fat, 80 mg sodium

113. **Best Specialty Meat**
Great Range Ground Bison
Make this lean, robust meat your new secret ingredient in Super Bowl party chili.
PER 4 OZ: 190 calories, 20 g protein,
0 g carbs, 11 g fat, 60 mg sodium

114. **Best Bacon**
Oscar Mayer Center Cut
Naturally Smoked
Don't fear bacon—it's low in calories. You need only a couple of strips to add flavor to potato salad, pizza, or soup.
PER 3 SLICES: 70 calories, 7 g protein, 0 g
carbs, 4.5 g fat, 270 mg sodium

115. **Best Sausage**
Al Fresco Sundried Tomato
Chicken Sausage with Basil and
Tomatoes
Split a link in half and broil it until the top begins to caramelize. Sprinkle with chopped cilantro and lime juice. Enjoy.
PER LINK: 140 calories, 15 g protein,
2 g carbs (0 g fiber, 2 g sugars),
7 g fat, 480 mg sodium

116. **Best Protein Powder**
At Large Nutrition
Nitrean Vanilla
A whey-casein blend that tastes good going down.
PER 30 G SCOOP: 113 calories, 23 g protein,
3 g carbs (N/A g fiber, N/A g sugars), 1 g fat,
95 mg sodium

COOKING STAPLES

117. **Best Hot Sauce**
Huy Fong Foods Tuong Ot Sriracha
Made from hot chilies, this sauce delivers a burn that enhances everything from scrambled eggs to chicken to salsa.
PER TBSP: 5 calories, 0 g protein,
1 g carbs (0 g fiber, 1 g sugars),
0 g fat, 100 mg sodium

118. **Best Everyday Oil**
Spectrum Organic Canola Oil
Its neutral taste is suitable for everyday cooking, and it has a well-balanced fatty acids profile, to help fight disease.
PER TBSP: 120 calories, 0 g protein,
0 g carbs, 14 g fat, 0 g sodium

119. Best High-End Olive Oil

Yellingbo Gold Extra
Virgin Olive Oil

This peppery, light-bodied oil tastes amazing drizzled on top of fresh pasta, mozzarella, or crusty bread.

PER TBSP: 120 calories, 0 g protein,
0 g carbs, 14 g fat, 0 mg sodium

120. Best Vinegar

Colavita Balsamic Vinegar

Mix ¼ cup of this with ½ cup of olive oil, chopped herbs, some shavings of Parmesan cheese (#21), salt, and pepper. Stir well for an easy vinaigrette.

PER TBSP: 15 calories, 0 g protein,
3 g carbs (0 g fiber, 3 g sugars),
0 g fat, 0 mg sodium

121. Best Salt

Maldon Sea Salt Flakes

This salt is perfect for heightening the flavors of fish, meat, or vegetables after they're cooked. Try it on a rib eye steak (#110) and taste the difference.
0 calories

122. Best Pepper

Simply Organic Whole
Black Peppercorns

Forget the pre-ground stuff in the shaker. Freshly ground pepper, combined with sea salt (#121), is the cornerstone of flavorful cooking. Use each to your taste.
0 calories

123. Best Bread Crumbs

Wel-Pac Japanese Style Panko
Bread Crumbs

A lighter, crunchier Japanese variety that's great sprinkled over sautéed string beans.

PER 28 G: 110 calories, 4 g protein,
20 carbs (1 g fiber, 1 g sugars), 1 g fat,
85 mg sodium

124. Best Low-Sodium Broth

Pacific Natural Foods
Organic Free-Range Chicken

Tastes like homemade, with far less sodium than most brands. Use it as a base for soups.

PER CUP: 15 calories, 2 g protein,
1 g carbs (0 g fiber, 0 g sugars),
0 g fat, 70 mg sodium

125. Best Soy Sauce

Kikkoman Less Sodium
Soy Sauce

Use it as a salt substitute in soups, marinades, and dressings to add a savory flavor to your meals.

PER TBSP: 10 calories, 1 g protein,
1 g carbs (0 g fiber, 0 g sugars),
0 g fat, 575 mg sodium

The Very Best Restaurant Foods

Cooking at home is almost always the best choice when it comes to keeping off the pounds. A University of Massachusetts study found that eating breakfast out instead of at home more than doubles your odds of obesity. Not only are restaurant meals often bigger than home-cooked ones, but you're also vulnerable to an impulse buy at a drive-thru or convenience store. Still, ya gotta get out once in a while. When you do, try this . . .

BREAKFAST

1. Best Oatmeal
Au Bon Pain Apple-Cinnamon Oatmeal (medium, 12 oz)
Between the rolled oats and apples, this bowl packs nearly a quarter of your day's recommended fiber without being overly sweet.
280 calories, 8 g protein, 56 g carbs
(7 g fiber, 14 g sugars), 4 g fat,
10 mg sodium

2. Best Breakfast Platter
Bob Evans Classic Breakfast
(two eggs, two bacon strips, and one slice of French toast)
The unfortunate truth about breakfast platters is that they're typically big enough to feed a small army. This one achieves the same combo effect without the belly-busting calorie load.
498 calories, 20 g protein, 20 g carbs
(1 g fiber, 11 g sugars), 33 g fat,
849 mg sodium

3. Best Breakfast Burrito
Carl's Jr. Bacon & Egg Burrito
Lighter breakfast burritos are out there, but if you want something sizeable enough to fill you up and substantial enough to pack a load of protein, this is the burrito for you.
550 calories, 29 g protein, 37 g carbs
(1 g fiber, 1 g sugars), 31 g fat,
970 mg sodium

4. Best Pancake Breakfast
Denny's Hearty Wheat Pancakes (stack of two)
Denny's fortifies its batter with wheat bran to make a fiber-rich stack of flapjacks that will to quell your hunger better than buttermilk pancakes ever could.
310 calories, 10 g protein, 64 g carbs
(8 g fiber, 2 g sugars), 1.5 g fat,
950 mg sodium

5. Best Waffle Breakfast

Bob Evans Belgian Waffle with Strawberry Topping

The lightest waffle you'll find at any fast-casual restaurant, and by choosing the strawberry topping over standard pancake syrup, you save almost 150 calories.

435 calories, 10 g protein, 75 carbs (4 g fiber, 29 g sugars), 10 g fat, 795 mg sodium

6. Best Doughnut

Dunkin' Donuts Sugar-Raised Donut

If you're craving an occasional doughnut, this one's your best bet—you won't find another with fewer than 200 calories.

230 calories, 3 g protein, 22 g carbs (1 g fiber, 4 g sugars), 14 g fat, 330 mg sodium

7. Best Filled Donut

Tim Hortons Strawberry-Filled Donut

The same strawberry-filled doughnut at Krispy Kreme carries twice the fat.

230 calories, 4 g protein, 36 g carbs (1 g fiber, 12 g sugars), 8 g fat, 220 mg sodium

8. Best Breakfast Pastry

Starbucks 8-Grain Roll

Starbucks might call this muffin-shaped breakfast bread a roll, but don't get confused: The protein and fiber counts make it a great way to start your morning.

350 calories, 10 g protein, 67 g carbs (5 g fiber, 17 g sugars), 8 g fat, 520 mg sodium

9. Best Cinnamon Roll

Krispy Kreme Cinnamon Bun

This cinnamon roll has a surprisingly low calorie count, especially compared with the Panera Bread version that clocks in with a walloping 620 calories.

260 calories, 3 g protein, 28 g carbs (< 1 fiber, 13 g sugars), 16 g fat, 125 mg sodium

10. Best Muffin

Starbucks Apple Bran Muffin

How do you pack 7 grams of fiber into a muffin? By including unrefined ingredients like whole-wheat flour and oats, along with apples, cherries, and cranberries.

350 calories, 6 g protein, 64 g carbs (7 g fiber, 34 g sugars), 9 g fat, 520 mg sodium

11. Best Croissant

Tim Hortons Plain Croissant

Croissants are always going to be high in saturated fat, so stick to the simplest variety and add a slice of ham for an extra hit of protein.

270 calories, 4 g protein, 23 g carbs (1 g fiber, 2 g sugars), 18 g fat, 210 mg sodium

12. Best Parfait

Bob Evans Blueberry-Banana Mini Fruit & Yogurt Parfait (6.7 oz)

Bob uses low-fat yogurt to minimize calories, and the bananas and blueberries on top deliver a healthy dose of fiber and antioxidants.

177 calories, 4 g protein, 39 g carbs (3 g fiber, 34 g sugars), 1 g fat, 61 mg sodium

13. **Best Breakfast Sandwich**
Subway Black Forest Ham, Egg, and Cheese Muffin Melt
Big hits of protein and fiber—not to mention an astonishingly low calorie count—make this the one of the best breakfast creations out there. Plus Subway offers something no other fast-food joint does: unlimited vegetables on your sandwich.
180 calories, 15 g protein, 18 g carbs (5 g fiber, 1 g sugars), 7 g fat, 650 mg sodium

14. **Best Breakfast Flatbread**
Dunkin' Donuts Egg White and Turkey-Sausage Flatbread
This sandwich boasts two sources of lean protein, egg whites and turkey sausage, so it's sure to fuel you all morning long.
290 calories, 21 g protein, 34 carbs (3 g fiber, 6 g sugars), 8 g fat, 600 mg sodium

15. **Best Whole-Egg Omelet**
Denny's Veggie-Cheese Omelette
An industry-wide reliance on butter and salt ensures that no restaurant-prepared omelet will ever compare with one made in your own kitchen. But you can minimize fat with a meatless variety—thanks to the cheese, you still get an extra helping of protein.
500 calories, 29 g protein, 10 g carbs (2 g fiber, 4 g sugars), 37 g fat, 940 mg sodium

16. **Best Egg-White Omelet**
Bob Evans Western Omelet with Egg Whites
Fully half of the calories in this vegetable-packed omelet come from protein.
300 calories, 37 g protein, 6 g carbs (1 g fiber, 2 g sugars), 14 g fat, 1,364 mg sodium

17. **Best Steak & Eggs**
Bob Evans Sirloin Steak and Two Farm-Fresh Eggs
The best way to keep a steak-and-eggs breakfast under control is by going with a lean cut of meat—such as sirloin—and having it seared.
683 calories, 47 g protein, 5 g carbs (0 g fiber, 2 g sugars), 51 g fat, 1,096 mg sodium

18. **Best Breakfast Potatoes**
Bob Evans Home Fries (5.1 oz serving)
Bob's reign over the breakfast landscape is official. These are the least-greasy spuds you'll ever wake up to.
164 calories, 3 g protein, 24 g carbs (3 g fiber, 0 g sugars), 6 g fat, 680 mg sodium

MEXICAN

19. **Best Drive-Thru Taco**
Del Taco Chicken Taco Del Carbon (two tacos)
A double layer of warm corn tortillas wrapped around chicken, chili sauce, cilantro, and diced onions make these tacos the closest to the authentic Mexican version you'll ever buy from a drive-thru window.
300 calories, 18 g protein, 38 g carbs (2 g fiber, 2 g sugars), 10 g fat, 600 mg sodium

20. **Best Sit-Down Taco**

Baja Fresh Original Baja Chicken Tacos (two tacos)

Too many Mexican restaurants use inauthentic flour tortillas and pack on the cheese. But Baja Fresh sticks to basics: corn tortillas, chicken, onions, cilantro, and salsa.

420 calories, 24 g protein, 56 g carbs (4 g fiber, N/A sugars), 10 g fat, 460 mg sodium

21. **Best Fish Taco**

Baja Fresh Grilled Mahimahi

Most taco-bound seafood is battered and fried. Shed the crust of fat by sticking to this grilled option.

460 calories, 24 g protein, 52 g carbs (8 g fiber, N/A sugars), 18 g fat, 600 mg sodium

22. **Best Burrito**

Taco Bell Supreme Steak Fresco Burrito

Taco Bell promotes this burrito by touting the fact that it has less than 9 grams of fat, but far more impressive are the 16 grams of protein and 8 grams of fiber that they've managed to cram inside.

330 calories, 16 g protein, 50 g carbs (8 g fiber, 4 g sugars), 8 g fat, 1,340 mg sodium

23. **Best Enchilada**

Chevys Salsa Chicken Enchiladas (two enchiladas)

Order these enchiladas à la carte with black beans on the side and you've just built one of the leanest entrees on Chevys menu.

460 calories, 30 g protein, 34 g carbs (4 g fiber, 6 g sugars), 22 g fat, 860 mg sodium

24. **Best Fajitas**

On the Border Mesquite-Grilled Chicken with El Diablo veggies, guacamole, pico de gallo, and three flour tortillas

You're not going to find a low-calorie plate of fajitas, but you can temper the damage by skipping the cheese, sour cream, and rice, which will save you 450 calories. The sodium count is still high, though, so you may want to split this with your dinner partner.

825 calories, 54 g protein, 74 g carbs (4 g fiber, N/A g sugars), 35 g fat, 1,960 mg sodium

25. **Best Taquitos**

Taco Bell Grilled Steak Taquitos (two taquitos)

The classic taquito is cooked in a hot vat of oil, but Taco Bell gets the job done with a flattop grill. That means far fewer calories from fat.

310 calories, 15 g protein, 37 g carbs, (2 g fiber, 3 g sugars), 11 g fat, 930 mg sodium

26. **Best Quesadilla**

El Pollo Loco Cheese Quesadilla

The same entrée at a sit-down restaurant will likely cost you more than 1,000 calories thanks to larger portion sizes and an excess of fillers.

420 calories, 19 g protein, 35 g carbs (2 g fiber, 0 g sugars), 23 g fat, 810 mg sodium

27. **Best Nachos**

Taco Bell Triple-Layer Nachos

The generous helping of beans on these nachos leaves less room for cheese and brings in a commendable dose of fiber.

350 calories, 7 g protein, 39 g carbs (7 g fiber, 2 g sugars), 18 g fat, 740 mg sodium

28. **Best Taco Salad**

Chipotle Barbacoa Salad Bowl
(lettuce, barbacoa, black beans,
guacamole, and green tomatillo
salsa; no vinaigrette)
*By opting for guacamole and salsa
instead of dressing, you add heart-
healthy monounsaturated fats and a
bevy of antioxidant-rich ingredients
from the salsa.*
465 calories, 35 g protein,
38 g carbs (19 g fiber, 5 g sugars), 21 g fat,
1,185 mg sodium

29. **Best Tortilla Soup**

El Pollo Loco Regular Chicken
Tortilla Soup with Tortilla Strips
(10.8 oz)
*Sodium is always an issue with torti-
lla soup, but El Pollo's recipe keeps
the damage minimal while still sup-
plying an impressive 16 grams of
protein.*
210 calories, 16 g protein, 18 g carbs
(2 g fiber, 2 g sugars), 9 g fat,
1,050 mg sodium

TRADITIONAL AMERICAN

30. **Best Steak**

Ruby Tuesday Plain-Grilled
Top Sirloin
*Avoid the extra 1,000 milligrams
of sodium that Ruby Tuesday uses
to season the regular sirloin by ordering this 9-ounce steak "plain"—the
restaurant's code word for "very little
salt."*
391 calories, 49 protein,
1 g carbs (0 g fiber, N/A sugars),
22 g fat, 1,456 mg sodium

31. **Best Smothered Steak**

Applebee's 9-oz House Sirloin
Topped with Sautéed Garlic
Mushrooms
*In restaurant-speak, "smothered"
often means a jumble of greasy vegetables and a layer of cheese. Sautéed
garlic and mushrooms are a much
better option.*
450 calories, 49 g protein, 1 g carbs
(0 g fiber, N/A sugars), 28 g fat,
1,190 mg sodium

32. **Best Ribs**

Ruby Tuesday Memphis
Dry-Rub Fork-Tender Ribs
(½ rack)
*Leaner ribs simply cannot be found.
At Outback Steakhouse, the half rack
has nearly three times as much fat.*
460 calories, 44 g protein,
6 g carbs (0 g fiber, N/A sugars), 29 g fat,
150 mg sodium

33. **Best Appetizer**

Ruby Tuesday Traditional Chicken
Strips (four strips)
*Being healthy doesn't mean skipping
a starter. Just make sure you order
these, which have the best nutritional
profile around.*
376 calories, N/A protein, 12 g carbs
(0 g fiber, N/A sugars), 16 g fat,
888 mg sodium

34. **Best Chicken Entrée**

Olive Garden Venetian
Apricot Chicken
*Chicken and vegetables offer the
perfect blend of protein and
carbohydrates, and Olive Garden's
tasty apricot citrus sauce is an
extra bonus.*
380 calories, N/A protein,
32 g carbs (8 g fiber, N/A sugars),
4 g fat, 1,420 mg sodium

35. **Best Barbecue Chicken**

Bob Evans Memphis Spice-Rubbed
Chicken Breast

The Memphis-style rub—with ingredients such as garlic, onion, and cayenne pepper—is a great way to get that barbeque taste without loading up on calories and sodium.

281 calories, 30 g protein, 17 g carbs
(1 g fiber, 15 g sugars), 10 g fat,
544 mg sodium

36. **Best Chicken Drumstick**

KFC Grilled Chicken
Drumsticks (two drumsticks)

We know it's not called Kentucky Grilled Chicken, but choosing Grilled Drumsticks over KFC's Original Drumsticks will save you 100 calories and 7 grams of fat. Thanks, Colonel.

160 calories, 22 g protein, 0 g carbs, 8 g fat,
460 mg sodium

37. **Best Chicken Nuggets**

Chic-fil-A Nuggets
(eight pieces)

Nugget for nugget, these chicken chunks have half as much fat as the McDonald's version.

270 calories, 28 g protein,
12 g carbs (1 g fiber, 2 g sugars), 12 g fat,
990 mg sodium

38. **Best Hot Dog**

Dairy Queen All-Beef Dog

When it comes to hot dogs, this one is as slim as they come. Practice prudence with the toppings and DQ's dog can be a fairly healthy protein-packed option.

290 calories, 11 g protein, 22 g carbs
(1 g fiber, 4 g sugars), 17 g fat,
900 mg sodium

39. **Best Chili-Cheese Dog**

Dairy Queen All-Beef
Chili-Cheese Dog

Consider this the most indulgent meal you'll ever find with fewer than 400 calories.

380 calories, 16 g protein, 23 g carbs
(1 g fiber, 3 g sugars), 24 g fat,
980 mg sodium

40. **Best Chili**

Wendy's Chili (small)

With an ample amount of fiber and protein in tow, Wendy's chili is one of our all-time favorite fast-food sides. Choose it instead of medium fries and you'll save nearly 200 calories while gaining a boost of cancer-fighting lycopene.

220 calories, 18 g protein,
22 g carbs (6 g fiber, 6 g sugars),
7 g fat, 870 mg sodium

41. **Best Bean Soup**

Au Bon Pain Split-Pea-and-Ham
(medium, 12 oz)

Fiber is a crucial element in the battle against unwanted weight gain, and this bowl of legumes has 50 percent of your day's recommended intake with a minor dose of fat.

250 calories, 18 g protein, 41 g carbs
(15 g fiber, 3 g sugars), 2 g fat,
1,220 mg sodium

42. **Best Chicken Noodle Soup**

Applebee's Chicken
Noodle Soup (bowl)

Commercially prepared soups are notoriously high in sodium, but at least this one boasts plenty of chicken to fill you up.

160 calories, 13 g protein,
17 g carbs (1 g fiber, N/A sugars), 4 g fat,
1,120 mg sodium

43. **Best Cheesy Soup**

Quiznos Broccoli-Cheese Soup (cup)
Some broccoli-and-cheese iterations are little more than a few florets floating in a sea of cheddar, so striking the proper balance between the two ingredients is crucial to your waistline. Just make sure you exercise portion control.
130 calories, 4 g protein, 9 g carbs
(1 g fiber, 2 g sugars), 9 g fat,
640 mg sodium

44. **Best Caesar Salad**

California Pizza Kitchen Classic Caesar with Grilled Shrimp
Upgrading the classic recipe with shrimp is a great way to inject lean protein, selenium, and vitamin D into your meal.
649 calories, 35 g protein,
30 g carbs (8 g fiber, N/A sugars),
15 g saturated fat, 1,338 mg sodium

45. **Best Fast-Food Meal**

Chick-fil-A Chargrilled Chicken Sandwich with Large Fruit Cup
How do you build the world's best fast-food meal? Pair the best sandwich with a cup of nutrient-rich fruit. That's an entire meal with fewer calories than most medium orders of french fries.
400 calories, 30 g protein, 65 g carbs
(6 g fiber, 32 g sugars), 3.5 g fat,
1,120 mg sodium

46. **Best Fast-Food Side**

Taco Bell Pintos 'N Cheese
The pinto beans in this cup happen to be one of the planet's healthiest foods. They're rich in fiber, antioxidants, and folate, a B vitamin with a strong link to weight loss. We'll take these over nachos any day.
170 calories, 10 g protein,
19 g carbs (9 g fiber, 1 g sugars), 6 g fat,
750 mg sodium

BURGERS AND SANDWICHES

47. **Best Fast-Food Burger**

McDonald's Big N' Tasty (no mayo)
Ordered sans mayo, the Big N' Tasty is without a doubt the leanest fast-food burger of its size.
410 calories, 24 g protein, 36 g carbs
(3 g fiber, 7 g sugars), 19 g fat,
640 mg sodium

48. **Best Sit-Down Restaurant Burger**

Red Robin Natural Burger
Most burgers have been embellished so much that they're barely recognizable beneath the excess layers of fat. This is one of the few that keeps it simple, clocking in under 600 calories.
569 calories, 37 g protein,
51 g carbs (3 g fiber, 9 g sugars),
24 g fat, 989 mg sodium

49. **Best Mushroom Burger**

Culver's Mushroom
& Swiss Single
*The law of burgers states that the
longer the name, the worse the burger
is for you. This one's an exception to
the rule.*
431 calories, 25 g protein, 33 g carbs
(1 g fiber, 5 g sugars), 20 g fat,
581 mg sodium

50. **Best Bacon Burger**

Five Guys Little Bacon Burger
*"Little" this burger most certainly is
not, but to the folks at Five Guys,
anything bigger than "little" amounts
to a double burger. So take the little
single—it's the biggest bacon burger
you'll find under 600 calories.*
560 calories, 27 g protein,
39 g carbs (2 g fiber, 8 g sugars), 33 g fat,
640 mg sodium

51. **Best Double Burger**

Wendy's Double Stack
*Thanks to a double portion of
Wendy's Jr. patties, this burger
keeps the calories low but the
meat-to-bun ratio high.*
360 calories, 23 g protein,
27 g carbs (1 g fiber, 6 g sugars),
18 g fat, 760 mg sodium

52. **Best Turkey Burger**

Red Robin Grilled
Turkey Burger
*Turkey burgers are generally no
healthier than their beef-based counterparts. (Many restaurants use
fattier turkey for a juicier burger.)
Order one at Ruby Tuesday, for
instance, and you're risking a
1,230-calorie backlash. This one's
much more reasonable.*
641 calories, 30 g protein,
50 g carbs (3 g fiber, 8 g sugars), 37 g fat,
1,000 mg sodium

53. **Best Veggie Burger**

Burger King BK Veggie Burger
*Of the big-three fast-food purveyors,
Burger King is the only one that offers
a veggie burger. And great news for
busy vegetarians: It trounces the
veggie offerings from all the major
sit-and-eat chains.*
400 calories, 22 g protein, 43 g carbs
(N/A fiber, 8 g sugars), 16 g fat,
1,020 mg sodium

54. **Best French Fries**

McDonald's French Fries (medium)
*You can find lower-calorie fries at
KFC and Dairy Queen, but both
chains still rely on partially hydrogenated oils to crisp their spuds.
Plus McD's fries have less than half
as much sodium.*
380 calories, 4 g protein, 48 g carbs
(5 g fiber, 0 g sugars), 19 g fat,
270 mg sodium

55. **Best Fried Onion**
Burger King Onion Rings (small)
The lowest-calorie rings we could find. Plus Burger King uses vegetable oil rather than trans-fatty partially hydrogenated oil.
310 calories, 4 g protein, 36 g carbs (3 g fiber, 4 g sugars), 17 g fat, 490 mg sodium

56. **Best Chicken Wings**
Pizza Hut WingStreet All-American Traditional Wings (five wings)
Hands down the lightest recipe when it comes to wings. Just make sure you order them "traditional" style. Ask for it "crispy" and you can expect nearly three times the fat.
400 calories, 35 g protein, 0 g carbs, 25 g fat, 1,450 mg sodium

57. **Best Roast Beef Sandwich**
Subway Roast Beef Sub (6-inch on 9-grain wheat bread)
Not only is this sandwich leaner than any of the roast-beef offerings at Arby's but you can also load it up with healthy vegetables.
310 calories, 26 g protein, 45 g carbs (5 g fiber, 6 g sugars), 4.5 g fat, 800 mg sodium

58. **Best Steak Sandwich**
Quiznos Roadhouse Steak Sammie
The bread used in the sammie is smaller than typical sandwich bread, which means more calories to spend on sautéed mushrooms, onions, and Quiznos' Sweet and Spicy Steak Sauce.
260 calories, 13 g protein, 38 g carbs (1 g fiber, 13 g sugars), 6 g fat, 980 mg sodium

59. **Best BLT**
Five Guys BLT (4 slices of bacon, lettuce, tomato, and mustard)
Even if you don't see a BLT on the menu, burger joints are equipped to put them together. Build your own at Five Guys and it'll be leaner than any burger the chain has to offer.
433 calories, 24 g protein, 42 g carbs (3 g fiber, 11 g sugars), 23 g fat, 911 mg sodium

60. **Best Reuben**
Schlotzsky's Small Angus Pastrami Reuben
The classic Reuben relies on a fat-packed triad of Thousand Island dressing, Swiss cheese, and corned beef. This version is the healthiest one you'll find with those ingredients.
618 calories, 41 g protein, 54 g carbs (4 g fiber, 4 g sugars), 26 g fat, 1,510 mg sodium

60. **Best Pulled Pork Sandwich**
White Castle Pulled Pork BBQ Sandwich (2)
This is as close to guilt-free as you can get with a pulled-pork BBQ sandwich. Even having three would be better than any other restaurant option.
340 calories, 18 g protein, 50 g carbs, (2 g fiber, 24 g sugars), 9 g fat, 920 mg sodium

62. **Best Ham and Cheese Sandwich**
Arby's Ham & Swiss Melt Sandwich
This warm, toasty sandwich satisfies despite its modest size.
300 calories, 18 g protein, 37 g carbs (2 g fiber, 6 g sugars), 8 g fat, 1,070 mg sodium

63. **Best Mini Sandwiches**

KFC Honey BBQ Snackers
(two sandwiches)

*For comparison, White Castle's
healthiest chicken sandwich carries
an extra 140 calories.*

420 calories, 26 g protein, 64 g carbs
(4 g fiber, 24 g sugars), 6 g fat,
940 mg sodium

64. **Best Grilled Chicken Sandwich**

Chic-fil-A Char-Grilled
Chicken Sandwich

*Low in calories and high in protein,
this sandwich is one of the fast-food
world's greatest achievements.
Pair it with a fruit cup for a perfectly
rounded lunch.*

300 calories, 29 g protein,
38 g carbs (3 g fiber, 10 g sugars),
3.5 g fat, 1,120 mg sodium

65. **Best Crispy Chicken Sandwich**

Wendy's Crispy Chicken Sandwich

*Wendy's manages what no other fast
food joint has been able to: Make
a crispy chicken sandwich with fewer
than 400 calories and less than
1,000 milligrams of sodium.*

350 calories, 15 g protein,
38 g carbs (2 g fiber, 4 g sugars), 15 g fat,
830 g sodium

66. **Best Chicken Salad Sandwich**

Atlanta Bread Company Chicken
Salad on Sourdough

*ABC's recipe bucks bad restaurant
habits by maintaining the proper
ratio of chicken to mayonnaise.*

440 calories, 29 g protein, 42 g carbs
(3 g fiber, 4 g sugars), 19 g fat,
680 mg sodium

67. **Best Classic Fish Sandwich**

McDonald's Filet-O-Fish

*There are two ingredients that,
when applied carelessly, can overpower the fish and sink the nutritional value: cheese and tartar sauce.
Thankfully, McDonald's applies
both with due prudence.*

380 calories, 15 g protein,
38 g carbs (2 g fiber, 5 g sugars), 18 g fat,
640 mg sodium

68. **Best Melt**

Arby's Melt

*Arby's roast beef has a peppery
tang that pairs perfectly with the
mellow flavor of Cheddar cheese.
And it's leaner than a burger.*

370 calories, 23 g protein, 40 g carbs
(2 g fiber, 6 g sugars), 13 g fat,
1,150 mg sodium

69. **Best Philly Cheesesteak**

Subway Big Philly Cheese-steak
(6-inch on 9-grain whole wheat)

*The sheer amount of beef makes
this one of the most filling sandwiches
on Subway's menu. And, thankfully,
it relies on real cheese instead of
Cheez Whiz.*

520 calories, 39 g protein,
53 g carbs (6 g fiber, 7 g sugars),
18 g fat, 1,570 mg sodium

70. **Best Veggie Sandwich**
Cosi Fire-Roasted Veggie Sandwich
Finally, there's a veggie sandwich that's more than just a garden salad between two pieces of bread. To deliver big flavor, Cosi brings in eggplant, roasted peppers, artichoke hearts, hummus, and feta, which helps bolster the protein count, too.
324 calories, 11 g protein,
44 g carbs (4 g fiber, 4 g sugars), 8 g fat,
259 mg sodium

71. **Best Wrap**
Dairy Queen Grilled
Chicken Wrap
Few restaurants seem able to make a chicken wrap without injecting a turkey baster's worth of mayonnaise. DQ manages otherwise. Sure, there's a touch of ranch sauce in this wrap, but it still adds up to a low calorie count.
200 calories, 12 g protein, 9 g carbs
(1 g fiber, 1 g sugars), 13 g fat,
450 mg sodium

ASIAN

72. **Best Dumplings**
P.F. Chang's Steamed Pork
Dumplings (six dumplings)
Ask for them steamed instead of pan-fried and cut 2 grams of fat from each dumpling.
360 calories, 24 g protein,
36 g carbs (0 g fiber, N/A sugars),
12 g fat, 750 mg sodium

73. **Best (two) Chinese Entrées**
Manchu Wok Beef and Broccoli
with Green Bean Chicken
The best Chinese entrée is actually two! But only if you order strategically. The usual approach at Chinese restaurants is to burden each plate with 300 to 450 calories of pure starch via noodles or rice. Skip those carbo-bombs and calories by ordering these two balanced entrées à la carte.
340 calories, 15 g protein, 22 g carbs
(4 g fiber, 8 g sugars), 23 g fat,
1,290 mg sodium

74. **Best Spicy Dish**
Panda Express Kung Pao Chicken
with Mixed Veggies
Kung Pao's peanuts deliver a nice package of metabolism-boosting B vitamins, and the mixed veggies sneak in some fiber, as well.
335 calories, 21 g protein,
21 g carbs (5 g fiber, 6 g sugars), 19 g fat,
1,140 mg sodium

75. **Best Pork Dish**
Manchu Wok BBQ Pork
with Mixed Vegetables
Pick this dish next time you need a dose of Chinese-style pork. The sweet-and-sour version carries more sugar and less protein.
370 calories, 24 g protein, 27 g carbs
(3 g fiber, 16 g sugars), 21 g fat,
1,240 mg sodium

76. **Best Side**

P.F. Chang's Spinach
Stir-Fried with Garlic (small)
*We always recommend replacing rice
and chow mein with more rewarding
ingredients, but rarely does Asian cuisine present the opportunity to enjoy
vitamin-rich spinach with your meal.*
80 calories, 6 g protein,
7.5 g carbs (4.5 g fiber, N/A sugars),
4.5 g fat, 450 mg sodium

77. **Best Spring Roll/or Egg Roll**

Manchu Wok Chicken
Egg Roll (one roll)
*With egg rolls, it's all about portion
control. These deep-fried torpedoes
can sink your chance of a healthy
meal, so stick with just one and keep
it around 150 calories.*
150 calories, 5 g protein, 17 g carbs
(1 g fiber, 1 g sugars), 7 g fat,
350 mg sodium

78. **Best Asian Soup**

Panda Express Egg Flower Soup
*This bowl manages two rare feats
in the soup world: It carries fewer
than 100 calories and has less than
1,000 milligrams of sodium.*
90 calories, 3 g protein,
15 g carbs (1 g fiber, 4 g sugars), 2 g fat,
810 mg sodium

79. **Best Asian Salad**

Panera Asian Sesame
Chicken Salad
*Most Asian salads suffer from an
overload of either sugar or sodium.
Panera's avoids both while emphasiz-
ing lean protein.*
400 calories, 31 g protein, 31 g carbs
(3 g fiber, 6 g sugars), 20 g fat,
810 mg sodium

ITALIAN

80. **Best Spaghetti**

Fazoli's Spaghetti or
Penne Marinara
*A modest amount of fat and antioxi-
dant-packed tomatoes make marinara the best sauce for any pasta dish.*
560 calories, 19 g protein, 111 carbs
(9 g fiber, 17 g sugars), 2.5 g fat,
970 mg sodium

81. **Best Alfredo**

Red Lobster Crab Linguine Alfredo
(lunch portion)
*Made from butter, Parmesan cheese,
and cream, Alfredo drowns pasta in
excess fat and sodium. Halve your
portion, toss in some protein for good
measure, and that's a meal well
managed.*
560 calories, N/A protein,
47 g carbs (N/A fiber, N/A sugars),
25 g fat, 1,310 mg sodium

82. **Best Stuffed Pasta**

Olive Garden's Ravioli di
Portobello (lunch portion)
*Low in sodium and a great source
of fiber, portobello mushrooms
are a delicious—and smart—way
to fill your ravioli and you.*
450 calories, N/A protein, 53 g carbs
(8 g fiber, N/A sugars), 19 g fat,
960 mg sodium

83. **Best Chicken Pasta**
Fazoli's Penne with Marinara, Broccoli, and Sliced Grilled Chicken
Fazoli's might be the fast food of Italian cuisine, but it's also the place that gives you the most control over your entrée. Keep it simple with a combo like this and you'll be better off.
695 calories, 39 g protein, 118 mg carbs (12 g fiber, 19 g sugars), 6 g fat, 1,490 mg sodium

84. **Best Lasagna**
Olive Garden's Lasagna Classico (lunch portion)
The full portion of this meal contains 2,830 milligrams of sodium and roughly one-third of your daily caloric intake. Lunch portions are an easy way to satisfy your craving without chaining you to the treadmill.
580 calories, N/A protein, 35 g carbs (7 g fiber, N/A sugars), 32 g fat, 1,930 mg sodium

85. **Best Parmesan**
Olive Garden Eggplant Parmigiana
The word "parmigiana" on a menu usually means trouble, but if you must, eggplant is a good source of fiber and will always save you calories over heavier options such as veal or chicken. Add a side of broccoli—the potassium will help balance the high sodium count.
850 calories, 98 g carbs (19 g fiber), 35 g fat, 1,900 mg sodium

86. **Best Italian Soup**
Culver's Minestrone (300 g)
Minestrone ingredients vary, but you can always depend on a bowl chock-full of vegetables, which keep the calorie count low while providing plenty of flavor and fiber.
100 calories, 4 g protein, 19 g carbs (4 g fiber, 4 g sugars), 1 g fat, 1,175 mg sodium

87. **Best Pizza**
Pizza Hut 12" Fit and Delicious, with Chicken, Mushrooms, and Jalapeño (two slices)
The Hut's Fit and Delicious line is by far the healthiest choice at any of the major pizza chains. Chicken, mushrooms, and jalapeños layer each slice with protein, a bit of fiber, and a touch of heat. Just make sure you exercise some discipline and stick to two slices.
340 calories, 22 g protein, 44 g carbs (2 g fiber, 8 g sugars), 9 g fat, 1,440 mg sodium

88. **Best Personal Pizza**
Pizza Hut Pepperoni and Mushroom Personal Pan Pizza
In this case, toppings are a good thing: Surprisingly, the plain cheese version has 20 extra calories.
570 calories, 24 g protein, 68 g carbs (4 g fiber, 7 g sugars), 23 g fat, 1,250 mg sodium

89. **Best Vegetarian Pizza**
Pizza Hut 12" Fit and Delicious, with Green Peppers, Red Onion, and Diced Red Tomato (two slices)
You save 100 calories compared to two slices of Pizza Hut's 12" Hand-Tossed Veggie Lover's.
300 calories, 12 g protein, 48 g carbs (4 g fiber, 10 g sugars), 8 g fat, 800 mg sodium

90. Best Flatbread

Uno Chicago Grill Roasted
Eggplant, Spinach, and Feta
($\frac{1}{2}$ flatbread)
*The feta's fat load is balanced with
a heavy hit of protein. Spinach and
eggplant only bring good energy to
this party, so fret not and enjoy.*
510 calories, 27 g protein,
58.5 g carbs (1.5 g fiber, 13.5 g sugars),
13 g fat, 990 mg sodium

SEAFOOD

91. Best Seafood Appetizer

Outback Seared Ahi Tuna (small)
*When it comes to appetizers—espe-
cially at Outback—this plate of
protein is a great way to start any
meal. Just don't go overboard with
the creamy ginger soy sauce and
wasabi vinaigrette dipping sauces.*
355 calories, 18.3 g protein, 11.5 g carbs
(2.2 g fiber), 23.3 g fat, 1,660 mg sodium

92. Best Fish Filet Entrée

Red Lobster Blackened Salmon
with Broccoli
*Salmon has an abundance of omega-
3s, which have been shown to reduce
your risk of heart disease. And since
the fish isn't smothered in creamy
sauce, the entrée is still low in fat.*
490 calories, 6 g carbs, 17 g fat,
440 mg sodium

93. Best Shrimp Entrée

Houlihan's Grilled Shrimp Entrée
with Panzanella Bread Salad
and Grilled Asparagus
*Shrimp is low in saturated fat and
high in protein—as long as it avoids
the deep fryer and fat-packed sauces.*
556 calories, 48 protein, 32 g carbs,
(5 g fiber), 26 g fat, 1,239 mg sodium

94. Best Breaded Fish

Red Lobster Fried Flounder
*Fish is a dish best served plain, but
if you prefer it fried, avoid the trans
fat by making sure the restaurant
doesn't use partially hydrogenated
oil. A light flaky fish such as flounder
will also help keep the calorie count
to a minimum.*
440 calories, N/A g protein, 5 g carbs,
16 g fat, 560 mg sodium

95. Best Crab Cakes

Long John Silver's Langostino
Lobster-Stuffed Crab Cake
*These decadent-sounding crab
cakes pack in plenty of seafood but
still boast a low calorie count.*
170 calories, 6 g protein, 1 g fiber,
9 g fat, 390 mg sodium

96. Best Shrimp Appetizer

Red Lobster Chilled
Jumbo Shrimp Cocktail
*You'd be hard-pressed to find
another appetizer that gives you this
much protein for so few calories.
Plus, shrimp is a great source of
selenium, an antioxidant that may
help prevent cancer.*
120 calories, N/A g protein, 9 g carbs
(N/A g fiber, N/A g sugars), 0.5 g fat,
580 mg sodium

97. Best Clam Chowder

Subway New England Clam
Chowder (10-oz bowl)
*Plenty of New England–style
clam chowders are heavy, but that
isn't a problem at Subway.*
150 calories, 6 g protein,
20 g carbs (4 g fiber, 2 g sugars), 5 g fat,
990 mg sodium

98. **Best Surf and Turf**
Red Lobster Wood-Grilled Peppercorn Sirloin with Steamed Snow Crab Legs
If you want to eat by land and by sea, snow crab legs and a modest portion of lean grilled steak are a great pair. The sodium count is high, though, so avoid the salt shaker for the rest of the day.
360 calories, N/A g protein, 0 g carbs, 10.5 g fat, 1,790 mg sodium

99. **Best Seafood Salad**
Macaroni Grill Scallops and Spinach Salad
Seared scallops will fill you up, and the fresh, wilted spinach provides a bevy of nutrients. Ask them to leave out the prosciutto to lower the sodium.
340 calories, 8 g protein, 11 g carbs (4 g fiber, N/A sugars), 31 g fat, 820 mg sodium

DESSERT

100. **Best Ice Cream**
Ben & Jerry's Scoop Shop Coffee Ice Cream (one scoop)
Just one scoop of ice cream can be a sugar land mine, especially when it's packed with swirls and bits of candy. This Ben & Jerry's flavor keeps the calories and sugar in check without being plain ol' vanilla.
190 calories, 3 g protein, 18 g carbs (0 g fiber, 16 g sugars), 11 g fat, 50 mg sodium

101. **Best Ice Cream Novelty**
Dairy Queen Ice Cream Sandwich
Somehow DQ has sandwiched ice cream between two chocolate wafers and made a treat that is no worse than a single scoop of ice cream. Don't ask questions; just be thankful.
190 calories, 4 g protein, 31 g carbs (1 g fiber, 18 g sugars), 5 g fat

102. **Best Ice Cream Topping**
Cold Stone Creamery Blueberries (15 g)
Blueberries are packed with antioxidants – and an intense hit of flavor. And since Cold Stone Creamery offers them as a healthy mix-in option, there's absolutely no need to add candy bar chunks to your ice cream.
10 calories, 0 g protein, 2 g carbs (0 g fiber, 2 g sugars), 0 g fat

103. **Best Frozen Yogurt**
Ben & Jerry's Vanilla Low-Fat Frozen Yogurt (one scoop)
Frozen yogurt carries less fat than ice cream, but to compensate, processors often jack up the sugar levels. This version is just the balance you're looking for.
130 calories, 4 g protein, 25 g carbs (0 g fiber, 16 g sugar), 1.5 g fat, 70 mg sodium

104. **Best Sorbet**
Macaroni Grill Italian Sorbetto
Made with lemons and raspberries, this dessert is a cool way to get your vitamin C fix.
150 calories, 0 g protein, 37 g carbs (0 g fiber, N/A sugars), 0 g fat, 5 mg sodium

105. **Best Ice**
Culver's Lemon Ice
(one scoop)
Ice and flavored syrup are all that goes into this summer-day salvation with a surprisingly modest amount of sugar.
84 calories, 0 g protein, 21 g carbs
(0 g fiber, 18 g sugars), 0 g fat,
4 g sodium

106. **Best Root Beer Float**
A&W Root Beer Float
(small, 16 oz)
No one does root beer better than A&W, and the same goes for floats. Ruby Tuesday's float, by comparison, has 169 extra calories and almost three times as much fat.
330 calories, 2 g protein,
70 g carbs (0 g fiber, 57 g sugars),
5 g fat, 100 mg sodium

107. **Best Sundae**
Uno Chicago Grill Mini Bananas
Foster (168 g)
Sure, there are sundaes with less fat and sugar, but do they come drizzled with a dose of rum? Nope. And since the portion size is under control, it's a smart indulgence.
350 calories, 4 g protein, 46 g carbs
(1 g fiber, 36 g sugars), 17 g fat,
140 mg sodium

108. **Best Brownie Sundae**
Uno Chicago Grill Mini Hot
Chocolate Brownie Sundae
A brownie sundae is basically two desserts in one. Uno's mini portion lets you enjoy the combo while avoiding a calorie crisis.
370 calories, 4 g protein,
54 g carbs (2 g fiber, 38 g sugars), 16 g fat,
1950 mg sodium

109. **Best Banana Split**
Sonic's Junior Banana Split (134 g)
Do you really need three helpings of ice cream in your banana split? Of course not. This one governs the heavy scooping and provides a dose of banana-based potassium.
210 calories, 2 g protein, 37 g carbs
(1 g fiber, 26 g sugars), 6 g fat,
90 mg sodium

110. **Best Cheesecake**
Schlotzky's New York–Style
Cheesecake (one slice)
Packed with cream cheese, cheesecake is often described as sinfully good, but a sinner you don't have to be. This slice from Schlotzky's has 315 fewer calories and 12 grams less saturated fat than Cheesecake Factory's Original Cheesecake.
350 calories, 6 g protein,
30 g carbs (1 g fiber, 19 g sugars),
23 g fat, 200 mg sodium

111. **Best Chocolate Cake**
Jack in the Box Chocolate
Overload Cake (one slice)
An intense hit of chocolate doesn't mean a mandatory overload of calories and fat. You'd be hard-pressed to find a better deal than this quick treat.
300 calories, 4 g protein, 57 g carbs
(2 g fiber, 34 g sugars), 7 g fat,
350 mg sodium

112. **Best Apple Pie**
McDonald's Baked Hot Apple Pie
More of a pocket than a traditional apple pie, but it's tasty and carries a modest amount of calories compared with other versions.
250 calories, 2 g protein, 32 g carbs
(4 g fiber, 13 g sugars), 13 g fat,
170 mg sodium

113. **Best Key Lime Pie**
Chili's Sweet Shot Key Lime Pie
Served in a shot glass, this is a
great alternative to ordering a whole
slice. Calories will add up fast if you
get a Sweet Shot Sampler, though, so
resist the urge.
240 calories, 4 g protein,
30 g carbs (0 g fiber, N/A sugars), 12 g fat,
75 mg sodium

DRINKS

114. **Best Coffee**
McDonald's Premium
Roast (small, 12 oz)
The confines of the dollar menu keep
it cheap, and the special blend of
Arabica beans keeps it rich. It's just
how a cup of joe should be.
0 calories

115. **Best Espresso Drink**
Starbucks Cappuccino with
2 Percent Milk (grande, 16 oz)
Choices abound at any coffee
shop, but the "simpler is better"
mantra applies here, too. A
cappuccino contains more froth
and less fluid milk than a latte,
which means fewer calories.
120 calories, 8 g protein, 12 g carbs
(0 g fiber, 10 g sugar), 4 g fat,
85 mg sodium

116. **Best Iced Coffee Drink**
Starbuck's Grande Iced Caffe
Americano (grande, 16 oz)
Starbuck's Iced Americano is just
a shot of espresso diluted with water
and served over ice, providing a
naturally subtle sweetness that
encourages a more sophisticated
coffee palate.
15 calories, <1 protein, 3 g carbs (0 g fiber,
0 g sugars), 0 g fat, 10 mg sodium

117. **Best Blended Coffee Drink**
Smoothie King Skinny Coffee
Smoothie Mocha (small, 20 oz)
Protein powder and nonfat milk make
this by far the best blended coffee
drink available.
260 calories, 17 g protein,
43 carbs (1 g fiber, 36 g sugars),
2 g fat, 226 mg sodium

118. **Best Hot Tea**
Jamba Juice Mighty Tea Leaf
Organic Green Dragon Tea
(16 oz)
Mighty Leaf uses premium green tea
from China and their roomy tea bags
allow the leaves to fully unfold,
maximizing the infusion process.
0 calories

119. **Best Sweetened Tea Drink**
Starbucks Tazo Shaken
Iced Green Tea (grande, 16 oz)
Specialty green tea drinks are all
the rage, but the best ones give
you a dose of antioxidants without
an excess of sugar. This Starbucks
drink does the trick.
80 calories, 0 g protein, 21 g carbs
(0 g fiber, 20 g sugars), 0 g fat,
10 mg sodium

120. **Best Fruit Smoothie**
Smoothie King Blueberry Heaven
(small, 20 oz)
*Like most smoothies, this version
is relatively high in sugar, but it
redeems itself with a helping of
protein and fiber. Just don't go
for the jumbo size.*
325 calories, 7 g protein, 73 g carbs
(2 g fiber, 64 g sugar), 1 g fat,
259 mg sodium

121. **Best Protein Smoothie**
Smoothie King High-Protein
Banana (20 oz)
*This smoothie is a great meal
replacer, low in calories but high
in protein. It also contains almonds,
which augment the protein count
while also offering heart-healthy
monounsaturated fats.*
322 calories, 27 g protein,
32 g carbs (4 g fiber, 23 g sugar), 9 g fat,
297 mg sodium

122. **Best Slush**
Sonic's Lemon Real Fruit Slush
(medium, 20 oz)
*Typically, slushes are a mixture
of ice and sugar-laden syrup.
Sonic's gets credit for bringing in
a touch of real fruit.*
290 calories, 0 g protein, 78 g carbs
(0 g fiber, 74 g sugars), 0 g fat,
45 mg sodium

123. **Best Cocktail**
Red Lobster Rob Roy
*Cocktails often include several
sugary mixers with an already sweet
liqueur. A Rob Roy keeps it simple
with scotch and sweet vermouth. Ask
for the drink with dry vermouth to
minimize your sugar intake.*
160 calories, N/A protein,
3 g carbs (N/A fiber, N/A sugars),
0 g fat, 10 mg sodium

124. **Best Margarita**
Olive Garden Wild Berry
Frozen Margarita
*The rare frozen margarita
under 300 calories.*
290 calories, N/A g protein
55 g carbs, (N/A g fiber, N/A g sugar)
0 g fat, 20 mg sodium

125. **Best Juice**
Jamba Juice Carrot Juice
(12 oz)
*A 12-ounce serving of this juice
provides 700 percent of your day's
vitamin A requirement plus shots of
both vitamin C and calcium in the
same number of calories as you'd find
in 8 ounces of Pepsi. The Pepsi,
however, scores nil for nutrients.*
100 calories, 3 g protein, 22 carbs
(0 g fiber, 20 g sugars), 0.5 g fat,
170 mg sodium

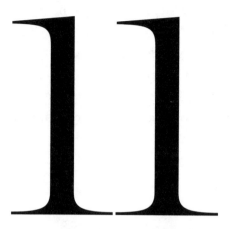

THE MEN'S HEALTH DIET RECIPES
MOUTHWATERING CONCOCTIONS TO FIGHT FAT AND FUEL YOUR MUSCLES.

The *Men's Health* Diet is designed to melt away pounds not by cutting down on the amount of food you eat, but by packing your day with nutrient-rich foods that are both filling and delicious. By following the *Men's Health* Diet Nutrition System, you'll strip away not only fat and useless calories, but also the unhealthy artificial compounds found in many processed foods that have been shown to contribute to weight gain. These recipes are quick and easy to follow. They'll help you crowd out unhealthy foods and additives because you'll stay full all day long as you burn calories easily and naturally—even while you sleep! And you'll feel healthier and happier, because The *Men's Health* Diet Nutrition System is designed to boost not only your body's fat-burning furnace, but also your brain's natural mood stabilizers.

The *Men's Health* Nutrition System
Breakfasts

Focus on eating a lot of calories in the forms of dairy, eggs, whole grains, and fiber

When you shift calories to the morning, you lose weight and keep it off. So eat a sizeable portion of your daily calories—30 to 35 percent of your total intake—in the morning. If you usually skip breakfast, you'll discover that you'll actually eat fewer calories throughout the day and gain less weight simply by eating 2 eggs and a slice of whole-grain toast every day. And if you have neither the time nor the stomach for a big breakfast first thing in the morning, try having two breakfasts—something small right after you get up, like a glass of milk and whole-wheat toast, and a larger breakfast or snack an hour or so later.

Pick-the-Lox Breakfast Burrito

2 Tbsp ricotta cheese

1 medium whole-wheat tortilla

1 oz smoked salmon, torn into little pieces

2 eggs, scrambled in a nonstick pan

1 cup baby spinach, chopped

1 green onion, sliced

Spread the cheese on the tortilla, then arrange the salmon, eggs, spinach, and green onions on top. Fold the ends in, roll, and enjoy.

Makes 1 serving. Per serving: *372 calories, 38 g protein, 25 g carbs (3 g fiber, 2 g sugars), 16 g fat, 477 mg cholesterol, 392 mg sodium*

Broccoli Spears Omelet

5 large eggs

half a fistful of fresh parsley, chopped

splash of soy sauce

2 tsp olive oil

2 Tbsp broccoli florets

5 spears asparagus, chopped

¼ cup string beans, halved

½ cup spinach

1 clove garlic, chopped

dash of black pepper

1. Mix the eggs, parsley, and soy sauce in a bowl.

2. Coat a skillet with the olive oil and sauté the broccoli, asparagus, beans, spinach, garlic, and black pepper for 5 minutes.

3. Pour the egg mixture over the vegetables. Stir it for about 30 seconds and then let it sit for 1 minute. Stir it again until the eggs firm up and then let it sit for another minute. Then fold it and remove it from the pan.

Makes 2 servings. Per serving: *223 calories, 15 g protein, 5 g carbs (2 g fiber, 2.5 g sugars), 14 g fat, 525 mg cholesterol, 172 mg sodium*

Nifty Quinoa Fruit Mash

1   **cup quinoa, rinsed**
2   **cups apple juice**
¼   **cup walnuts, crushed**
1   **cup organic berries**
     dash of cinnamon
3   **mint leaves**

1. In a saucepan, bring the quinoa and apple juice to a boil and then lower the heat to a simmer.

2. Cover and cook for 15 minutes until the quinoa is translucent.

3. Remove the pan from the heat and let the quinoa rest, covered, for 2 minutes. Put it into a bowl and stir in the nuts, berries, cinnamon, and mint.

Makes 2 servings. Per serving: *367 calories, 7 g protein, 62 g carbs (6 g fiber, 35 g sugars), 12 g fat, 0 mg cholesterol, 15 mg sodium*

Cream of the Crop

½   **cup evaporated milk**
2   **Tbsp whole-grain Cream of Wheat cereal or Wheatena**
1   **Tbsp flaxseed, ground**
½   **tsp vanilla extract**
1   **Tbsp walnuts, chopped**
1   **tsp maple syrup**
1   **Tbsp dried cranberries**

1. Combine the milk and cereal in a microwaveable bowl or mixing cup. Whisk with a fork. Microwave on high power for 2 minutes. Whisk again. Microwave in 30-second intervals, whisking after each interval, for about 60 seconds or until thickened. Stir in the flaxseed and vanilla extract. Spoon into a cereal bowl. Set aside.

2. Coat a small microwaveable plate with cooking spray. Spread the walnuts on the plate. Drizzle them with syrup. Microwave on high power for about 45 seconds or until sizzling. Using a spatula, scatter the glazed walnuts over the cereal mixture. Top with the cranberries.

Makes 1 serving. Per serving: *370 calories, 14 g protein, 44 g carbs (5 g fiber, 21 g sugars), 16 g fat, 35 mg cholesterol, 140 mg sodium*

Tortilla Flat Belly

5   soft corn tortillas (6" diameter)

6   scallions, chopped

1   red bell pepper, chopped

1   small jalapeño pepper, seeded and finely chopped (optional)

1   clove garlic, minced

1   tsp ground cumin

1   can (15 oz) reduced-sodium black beans, rinsed and drained

4   cups (about 4 oz) baby spinach

1   large tomato, chopped

1   cup Cheddar cheese, shredded

4   Tbsp sour cream

    fresh cilantro, chopped, for garnish

1. Preheat the oven to 350°F. Stack the tortillas on a large piece of foil, sprinkle the top one with water, and wrap them in the foil. Heat for 10 minutes.

2. Meanwhile, heat a large skillet coated with olive oil cooking spray over medium-high heat. Add the scallions and bell pepper and cook for 5 minutes, or until lightly browned. Add the jalapeño pepper (if using), garlic, and cumin. Cook for 2 minutes or until lightly browned. Stir in the beans, spinach, and tomato. Cook for 2 minutes or until heated through. Spread the mixture evenly in the skillet.

3. Remove the mixture from the heat and sprinkle it with the cheese. Let it stand until the cheese is melted. Top with dollops of sour cream and sprinkle it with the cilantro.

4. Cut the warmed tortillas into quarters or strips. Serve immediately with the cheesy bean-vegetable mixture.

Makes 4 servings. Per serving: *275 calories, 14 g protein, 30 g carbs (9 g fiber, 4 g sugars), 13 g fat, 35 mg cholesterol, 446 mg sodium*

Cluck, Moo and Oink Sandwich

1   slice (1 oz) bacon
½   tsp extra-virgin olive oil
1   egg
1   multigrain English muffin, toasted
1   oz (about 1 cup, packed) trimmed spinach leaves or baby spinach
½   freshly ground black pepper
1   slice Swiss, Jarlsberg, or Havarti cheese

1. Cook bacon slice per package directions.

2. Heat the oil in a small skillet over medium heat. Add the egg and heat it until the edges begin to set, about 1 minute. Lift the edges to allow any uncooked egg to flow underneath. When it's almost set, gently flip the egg. Cook another minute, then transfer to the bottom half of the muffin and top with the bacon.

3. Return the pan to the heat, add the spinach, and cook, stirring until it's wilted, about 1 minute. Place the spinach on top of the bacon, season with the pepper, add the cheese, and top with the other muffin half.

Makes 1 serving. Per serving (computed with Swiss cheese):
270 g calories, 20 g protein, 28 g carbs (6 g fiber, 2 g sugars), 12 g fat, 20 mg cholesterol, 200 mg sodium

Have a Pita on Me!

4   white mushrooms, sliced
1   Tbsp onion, chopped
1   Tbsp red bell pepper, chopped
     pinch of ground black pepper
2   eggs
½   small tomato, seeded and chopped
3   Tbsp milk
1   whole-wheat pita, halved and toasted
½   avocado, sliced

1. Coat a skillet with olive oil cooking spray and place over medium heat. Add the mush-rooms, onion, bell pepper, and black pepper. Cook for 3 to 4 minutes.

2. Meanwhile, in a bowl, combine the eggs, tomato, and milk. Whisk together until frothy. Pour the egg mixture into the skillet. Cook, stirring, for 3 to 4 minutes, or until the eggs are firm.

3. Fill each pita with half the eggs and top with the avocado slices.

Makes 1 serving. Per serving: *436 calories, 22 g protein, 40 g carbs (9 g fiber, 7 g sugars), 23 g fat, 428 mg cholesterol, 411 mg sodium*

Seeds of Contentment

6 cups old-fashioned oats, preferably thick-cut

1¼ cups raw almonds, sliced

1 package (7 oz) dried fruit bits

1 cup toasted wheat germ

½ cup unsalted raw pumpkin seeds

½ cup unsalted raw sunflower seeds

1. Preheat the oven to 325°F.

2. Spread the oats on a baking pan. Spread the almonds in a separate small baking pan. Place the oats and almonds in the oven and bake, stirring often, until the oats are lightly browned and the almonds are toasted. The oats will take 30 to 35 minutes; the almonds will toast in 20 to 25 minutes.

3. Place the oats and almonds in a large bowl and cool completely.

4. Add the fruit bits, wheat germ, pumpkin seeds, and sunflower seeds. Toss to combine. Store in an airtight container.

5. Serve with organic milk or yogurt.

Makes 22 servings. Per serving: *190 calories, 7 g protein, 26 g carbs (4 g fiber, 7 g sugars), 6.5 g fat, 0 mg cholesterol, 11 mg sodium*

The *Men's Health* Nutrition System
Lunches

Focus on vegetables, beans, fruits, nuts, and whole grains

Lunch is a pit stop to allow you to take on the fuel you need to power through the afternoon. Aim for at least 3 servings of vegetables—which are mainly water, fiber, and vitamins, so they will keep you hydrated and full with healthy calories.

My Chicken Can Dance the Salsa

1   tsp canola oil
2   corn tortillas (6" diameter)
     avocado, sliced
1   oz skinless chicken breast, cooked and thinly sliced
1   leaf lettuce, shredded
2   tsp store-bought salsa
2   tsp fresh cilantro, minced

1. Heat the oil in a skillet over medium-high heat. Cook the tortillas for about 1 minute on each side, or until lightly browned (they will become crisp as they cool).

2. Transfer the tortillas to a work surface. Place the avocado on 1 tortilla. Top it with the chicken, lettuce, salsa, cilantro, and remaining tortilla.

3. With a serrated knife, cut it into 2 half-moons.

Makes 1 serving. Per serving: *264.5 calories, 13 g protein, 27 g carbs (6 g fiber, 1 g sugars), 13 g fat, 24 mg cholesterol, 112 mg sodium*

Orange Ya Glad I Made Sweet Potato Salad?

2   large sweet potatoes (about 1¼ lb), peeled and cut into 1" cubes
4   Tbsp olive oil
1   tsp salt
2   thick slices bacon (2 oz total)
1   red bell pepper, chopped
1   small red onion, halved and thinly sliced
1   Tbsp fresh ginger, minced
1   tsp ground cumin
⅓   cup orange juice (1 orange)
1   lb fresh spinach leaves
    freshly ground black pepper, to taste
    pinch of salt (optional)

1. Heat oven to 400°F. Put the sweet potatoes on a baking sheet, drizzle them with 2 tablespoons of the oil, sprinkle with ¾ teaspoon of the salt, and toss to coat. Roast, turning occasionally, until crisp and brown on the outside and just tender inside, about 30 minutes. Remove them from the oven but leave them on the pan until ready to use.

2. While the potatoes roast, cook the bacon in a skillet over medium heat turning once or twice, until crisp. Drain the bacon on paper towels and pour off the fat, leaving any darkened bits in the pan. Chop the bacon. Put pan back over medium heat and add the remaining 2 tablespoons of oil. When hot, add the bell pepper, onion, ginger, and remaining ¼ teaspoon salt. Cook, stirring once or twice, until no longer raw. Stir in the cumin and bacon. Stir in the orange juice and turn off heat.

3. Put the spinach in a large bowl. Add the sweet potatoes, the warm dressing, and the freshly ground black pepper, to taste, and toss to combine. Taste and add salt if needed.

Makes 4 servings. Per serving: *274 calories, 7 g protein, 28 g carbs (6 g fiber, 10 g sugars), 16 g fat, 4 mg cholesterol, 799 mg sodium*

Smokin' Trout Salad

¾ lb golden beets, unpeeled, rinsed

2 Tbsp extra-virgin olive oil

3½ tsp lemon juice

2 tsp yuzu juice (available through gourmet Web sites, or you can use lime juice)

½ tsp salt

1 bunch watercress, thick stems trimmed

2 endives, halved lengthwise and thinly sliced crosswise

2 Asian pears, cut into ½"-thick wedges

1 (8 oz) smoked trout, skin and bones removed, cut into 8 pieces

1. Preheat the oven to 400°F. Wrap the beets in foil and place them on a baking sheet. Roast them for 1 hour and 15 minutes, or until the package yields to gentle pressure. When the beets are cool enough to handle, slip off the skins and cut them into thin wedges.

2. In a large bowl, whisk together the oil, lemon juice, yuzu juice, and salt. Add the watercress, endives, and Asian pears, and toss to coat.

3. Divide the salad among four plates and top with the beets and trout.

Makes 4 servings. Per serving: *304 calories, 22 g protein, 32.5 g carbs (15.5 g fiber, 16 g sugars), 11 g fat, 80.5 mg cholesterol, 430 mg sodium*

Vegetarian Curry Burgers

2   Tbsp olive or canola oil

1   medium onion, chopped (about 1 cup)

1   tsp curry powder

½   tsp ground coriander

½   tsp crushed fennel seeds

1½ cups white button mushrooms, chopped

1   cups chickpeas, cooked and drained

1   medium carrot, grated (about 1 cup)

¼   cup walnuts, chopped

3   Tbsp cilantro, chopped

½   tsp salt

¼   tsp ground black pepper
    flour

1. In a medium skillet over medium-high heat, warm 1 tablespoon of the oil.

2. Add the onion, curry powder, coriander, and fennel seeds. Cook, stirring frequently, for about 2 minutes, or until the onion starts to soften.

3. Add the mushrooms. Stir to mix. Cover and cook for about 4 minutes longer, or until the liquid pools in the pan.

4. Uncover and cook for about 3 minutes more, or until the liquid is evaporated.

5. Transfer the mixture to the bowl of a food processor fitted with a metal blade. Add the chickpeas. Pulse until well chopped. Transfer to a bowl.

6. Add the carrot, walnuts, cilantro, salt, and pepper to the bowl and mix well.

7. Lightly dust hands with flour. Shape the mixture into six 4"-wide patties.

8. In a large skillet over medium heat, warm the remaining 1 tablespoon of oil. Place the patties in the pan. Cook them for about 4 minutes, or until browned on the bottom. Flip them and cook for about 4 minutes longer or until heated through. Top them and serve them as you would any burger.

Makes 6 burgers. Per serving : *170 calories, 6 g protein, 18 g carbs (5 g fiber, 4 g sugars), 9 g fat, 0 mg cholesterol, 18 mg sodium*

Pushed 'n' Pulled Pork

1   tsp salt
1   tsp paprika
1   tsp chili powder
½   tsp ground cumin
⅛   tsp cayenne
4   lb bone-in pork shoulder, cut into 3 pieces and trimmed of all visible fat
1   onion, thinly sliced
½   cup brown sugar
½   cup ketchup
⅓   cup cider vinegar
¼   cup tomato paste
¼   cup water
2   Tbsp mustard
2   Tbsp Worcestershire sauce
½   tsp hot-pepper sauce

1. Mix the salt, paprika, chili powder, cumin, and cayenne. Rub the mixture over the pork.

2.Combine the pork and the onion, brown sugar, ketchup, cider vinegar, tomato paste, water, mustard, worcestershire sauce, and hot-pepper sauce in a large slow cooker. Cover and cook on low for 6 to 8 hours.

3. Remove the pork from the slow cooker and discard the bone. Cool for 10 minutes.

4. Using forks, shred the pork. Combine the pork with the sauce from the cooker. Serve over a toasted English muffin or hamburger bun.

Makes 12 servings. Per serving: *282 calories, 30 g protein, 14 g carbs (1 g fiber, 13 g sugars), 11 g fat, 101 mg cholesterol, 530 mg sodium*

Grilled Fish and White Bean Salad

2   Tbsp extra-virgin olive oil
2   Tbsp lemon juice
1   tsp grated lemon zest
    pinch of coarse salt
    pinch of pepper
1½ cups skinless salmon or
    tuna pieces, grilled and
    broken into large chunks
2   cups cooked white beans
1   cup cooked green beans
1   cup grape tomatoes, halved
⅓   cup red onion, thinly sliced
1½ tsp fresh sage, thinly
    shredded, or rosemary
    leaves, minced

1. In a large bowl, whisk together the oil, lemon juice, lemon zest, salt, and pepper. Measure out 1 tablespoon of the dressing and toss it with the fish in a medium bowl.

2. In a large bowl, toss the remaining dressing with the white beans, green beans, tomatoes, onion, and sage or rosemary.

3. Divide the vegetable mixture among 4 plates and top with the fish. Serve at room temperature or chilled.

Makes 4 servings. Per serving: *374 calories, 32 g protein, 31 g carbs (8.5 g fiber, 3 g sugars), 14 g fat, 60 mg cholesterol, 116 mg sodium*

6 Degrees of Kale 'n' Bacon

3 slices bacon, finely chopped

1 Tbsp olive oil

1 medium onion, finely chopped

4 cloves garlic, minced

4 cups chicken broth

4 cups cooked cannellini beans

1 small sprig fresh rosemary

1 sprig fresh sage

3 cups kale, finely chopped

salt and pepper, to taste

1. In a heavy-bottomed soup pot, cook the bacon over medium heat until the fat has rendered and the bacon is crisp, 10 to 12 minutes.

2. Add the olive oil, increase the heat to medium-high, and toss in the onion and garlic. Cook until the onion is softened and translucent, 5 to 7 minutes.

3. Add the broth, beans, rosemary, and sage and bring to a boil. Reduce the heat to medium-low and simmer for 15 minutes. Remove and discard the rosemary and sage.

4. Transfer half of the solids to a food processor or blender and combine until smooth.

5. Return the blended mixture to the soup pot and stir to combine. Bring the soup back to a quick boil, remove the pot from the heat, and add the kale. Season to taste with salt and pepper.

Makes 6 servings. Per serving: *291 calories, 18 g protein, 38 g carbs (9 g fiber, 1 g sugars), 9 g fat, 8 mg cholesterol, 214 mg sodium*

Too Good to Be Called "Salad"

2 salmon fillets (6 oz each), rinsed and dried

1 tsp dried or fresh parsley

juice of ½ lemon

1 tsp ground black pepper + 1 pinch

4 cups spinach leaves

10 grape or cherry tomatoes, halved

½ cup blueberries

1 tsp extra-virgin olive oil

½ cup sweet onion, chopped

1 clove garlic, minced

20 asparagus spears, bottoms cut off

½ yellow bell pepper, cut into strips

1 Tbsp honey mustard (use the lowest-sodium one you can find)

1 Tsbp almonds, slivered

1. Place the salmon in a deep skillet big enough for the salmon to lie flat on the bottom. Cover the fish with 1" of water.

2. Add the parsley, lemon juice, and 1 teaspoon of black pepper.

3. Bring to a boil over medium heat. Boil for 10 to 15 minutes, or until the fish is opaque.

4. Lightly scrape off the skin and fat line.

5. Evenly divide the spinach, tomato, and blueberries between two plates. Top each with half of the salmon.

6. In another skillet, combine the oil, onion, and garlic. Cook over medium-high heat for 2 minutes, or until lightly browned.

7. Add the asparagus, bell pepper, and a pinch of black pepper.

8. Reduce the heat to medium. Cook for 2 to 3 minutes, or until the veggies are slightly tender.

9. Add the honey mustard. Cook for 30 seconds longer, or until the honey mustard slightly caramelizes.

10. Place the mixture over the salmon. Sprinkle with the almonds.

Makes 2 servings. Per serving: *496 calories, 42 g protein, 33 g carbs (10 g fiber, 13 g sugars), 23 g fat, 100 mg cholesterol, 238 mg sodium*

The *Men's Health*
Nutrition System
Dinners

Focus on leafy greens and other vegetables, lean meats,
fish, beans, and other legumes

Studies show that if you start your dinner with a small side green salad dressed with olive oil and vinegar or with steamed folate-rich vegetables like kale, spinach, collard greens, and Swiss chard, you'll decrease your overall food intake by 12 percent while taking in satiating fiber and disease-fighting nutrients. Plus, folate-rich greens will give you a mood boost.

Holy Mackerel!

½   cup olive oil
1   Tbsp Dijon mustard
      juice of 2 lemons
      handful of fresh parsley
2   mackerel fillets
      salt and pepper, to taste
2   cups kale

1. Whisk together the olive oil and the Dijon mustard, the lemon juice, and the parsley.

2. Season the mackerel fillets with salt and pepper and a spoonful of the vinaigrette. Cook them over medium heat on a clean, oiled grill for 3 to 4 minutes a side until they're lightly charred and firm to the touch.

3. While the fish is cooking, quickly steam the kale.

4. Combine the fish and kale and drizzle on plenty of vinaigrette before serving.

Makes 2 servings. Per serving: *347 calories, 25.5 g protein, 33 g carbs (8 g fiber, 1 g sugars), 14 g fat, 93 mg cholesterol, 161 mg sodium*

Sage-Crusted Chicken Tenders and Crispy Kale Chips

CHICKEN TENDERS

1   egg white
1   Tbsp sesame seeds
1   Tbsp finely chopped sun-flower seeds
¾   tsp finely chopped sage
⅛   tsp freshly ground black pepper
2   boneless, skinless chicken tenders (2 oz each)
1   Tbsp spicy brown mustard
1   tsp honey

KALE CHIPS

1½ cups packed kale, cut into 1½" pieces
1   tsp garlic, minced
1   tsp extra-virgin olive oil
½   tsp sesame seeds
    salt and freshly ground pepper, to taste

1. Preheat the oven to 400°F. Coat a baking sheet with canola oil cooking spray. Place the egg white in a shallow bowl. Combine half of the sesame seeds, sunflower seeds, sage, and pepper in another small bowl.

2. Using a fork, dip the chicken in the egg white to coat both sides, then dip them in the sesame seed mixture, coating both sides.

3. Transfer to one half of the baking sheet and mist the chicken with cooking spray. Flip the chicken with a fork and mist the other side.

4. Combine the kale, garlic, oil, and other half of the sesame seeds in a medium bowl, tossing to coat. Season with salt and freshly ground black pepper. Transfer the kale to the other half of the baking sheet. (Note: The kale does not need to be in a single layer.)

5. Bake for 15 to 17 minutes, or until the chicken is cooked through and the kale is crisp and the edges are browned. Flip the chicken and toss the kale halfway through the cooking time.

6. Combine the mustard and honey in a small bowl and serve as a dipping sauce for the chicken tenders.

Makes 1 serving. Per serving: *385 calories, 37 g protein, 22 g carbs (4.5 g fiber, 6 g sugars), 16 g fat, 66 mg cholesterol, 324 mg sodium*

Feel-the-Heat Fajitas

1¼ lb boneless pork loin chops, trimmed and sliced into ½" strips

grated peel and juice of 1 lime

3 cloves garlic, minced

½ tsp kosher salt

¼ tsp cayenne pepper

¼ tsp ground black pepper

4 tsp + 1 Tbsp canola oil

3 large bell peppers (mixed colors), seeded and cut into long, ½"-thick strips

1 extra-large onion, cut into ½"-thick slices

2 jalapeño peppers, seeded and cut into thin strips, wear plastic gloves when handling

1 cup cilantro leaves, tough stems discarded and loosely packed

12 6" flour tortillas, warmed

1. Place the pork in a bowl with the lime zest, half of the lime juice, the garlic, salt, cayenne, black pepper, and 2 teaspoons of the oil. Toss to coat. Marinate the pork at room temperature for 20 minutes (or longer, or overnight in the fridge).

2. Heat 1 tablespoon of oil in a wok (or 12-inch skillet) over medium-high heat. Add the bell peppers, onion, and jalapeño. Stir-fry until the onions and peppers are soft and slightly charred, 6 to 8 minutes. Transfer the peppers and onions to a metal bowl and toss with cilantro and the remaining lime juice. Cover with foil and keep warm.

3. Return the wok to medium-high heat. Add the remaining 2 teaspoons of oil and the pork. Stir-fry until the meat is seared and just cooked through, 3 to 4 minutes. Place the pork in warmed tortillas and top with the vegetables.

Makes 6 servings. Per serving: *521 calories, 29 g protein, 58 g carbs (5 g fiber, 6 g sugars), 19 g fat, 60 mg cholesterol, 837 mg sodium*

Scallops on a Gallop

2 strips bacon, chopped into small pieces

½ red onion, minced

1 clove garlic, minced

1½ cans white beans (14 oz each), rinsed and drained

4 cups baby spinach

1 lb large sea scallops
salt and pepper, to taste

1 Tbsp butter
juice of 1 lemon

1. Heat a medium saucepan on low and cook the bacon until it begins to crisp. Pour off some of the bacon fat and add the onion and garlic. Sauté until the onion is soft and translucent, about 2 to 3 minutes. Add the beans and spinach. Cook until the beans are hot and the spinach is wilted. Keep warm.

2. Heat a large cast-iron skillet or sauté pan on medium-high. Blot the scallops dry with a paper towel and season them on both sides with salt and pepper. Add the butter to the pan. After it melts, add the scallops. Sear them for 2 to 3 minutes on each side until they're deeply caramelized.

3. Before serving, add the lemon juice to the beans, along with some salt and pepper. Divide the beans among four warm bowls or plates and top them with the scallops.

Makes 4 servings. Per serving: *284 calories, 28 g protein, 28 g carbs (7 g fiber, 2 g sugars), 7 g fat, 50 mg cholesterol, 400 mg sodium*

Black & White Stir Fry

STIR-FRY SEASONING

2   Tbsp dried onion

2   Tbsp garlic powder

2   tsp dried parsley

½   tsp ground ginger

¼   tsp crushed red-pepper flakes

½   tsp salt

STIR-FRY

2   tsp olive oil

2   medium red bell pepper, chopped

1   small onion, chopped

1   small zucchini, halved and cut into chunks

2   cloves garlic, minced

1   bag (16 oz) shirataki noodles, drained and rinsed in hot water

1   cup canned black beans, drained and rinsed

2   Tbsp reduced-sodium soy sauce

2   Tbsp fresh cilantro, chopped

    hot-pepper sauce

1. In a small bowl, combine the dried onion, garlic powder, parsley, ginger, red-pepper flakes, and salt.

2. Warm the oil in a wok or large cast-iron skillet over high heat. Add the bell peppers, onion, zucchini, and garlic. Reduce the heat to medium-high and cook, stirring frequently, for 4 minutes or until the vegetables start to soften.

3. Add the noodles, beans, soy sauce, and seasoning mix. Reduce the heat to medium. Cook, stirring frequently, for 3 to 4 minutes longer, or until the mixture is hot. Add the cilantro. Toss to mix.

4. Season with hot-pepper sauce to taste at the table.

Makes 4 servings. Per serving: *106.5 calories, 5 g protein, 18 g carbs 5 g fiber, 4 g sugars), 3 g fat, 0 mg cholesterol, 538.5 mg sodium*

I Just Feta Chicken

2   **Tbsp jarred sun-dried tomatoes, chopped**

2   **Tbsp feta cheese, crumbled**

2   **Tbsp olives, chopped**

2   **garlic cloves, minced**

1   **Tbsp balsamic vinegar**

2   **free-range organic chicken breasts**

    extra-virgin olive oil

    salt and black pepper, to taste

2   **cups organic spinach**

1. Preheat the oven to 450°F. Toss together the tomatoes, feta cheese, olives, 1 clove of minced garlic, and vinegar.

2. Rub the chicken with olive oil, salt, and pepper. Using a small, sharp knife, carefully cut a slit along the thick part of each chicken breast, creating a pocket. Add enough tomato mixture to fill each pocket and transfer the chicken to a baking sheet.

3. Bake for about 15 minutes, until the chicken juices run clear. Top with any remaining stuffing.

4. While chicken is cooking, sauté the spinach with the remaining tablespoon of olive oil and minced garlic clove. Serve alongside the chicken.

Makes 2 servings. Per serving: *634 calories, 60 g protein, 29 g carbs (2 g fiber, 4 g sugars), 29 g fat, 153 mg cholesterol, 791 mg sodium,*

Red-Headed Burritos

10 dry-packed sun-dried tomatoes

1 cup boiling water + 2½ cups water

1 cup dry red lentils, sorted and rinsed

1 Tbsp olive oil

½ cup onions, chopped

½ cup broccoli florets, chopped

½ cup cauliflower florets, chopped

½ cup carrots, thinly sliced

1½ cups tomato sauce

1 tsp curry powder

½ tsp ground cinnamon

4 whole-wheat tortillas (8" diameter), warmed

1. Place the sun-dried tomatoes in a small bowl and cover with the boiling water. Let soak for 10 minutes, or until the tomatoes are soft. Drain, reserving ½ cup of the soaking liquid.

2. Chop the tomatoes and set aside.

3. In a medium saucepan, combine 2½ cups of water, the lentils, and the reserved soaking liquid. Bring to a boil over medium-high heat. Reduce the heat to low and simmer for 6 to 10 minutes, or just until the lentils are tender. Drain and set aside.

4. In a large cast-iron or stainless steel skillet over medium heat, warm the oil. Add the onions, broccoli, cauliflower, and carrots. Sauté for 4 to 5 minutes or until the vegetables are tender. Stir in the tomato sauce, curry powder, and cinnamon. Add the lentils and sun-dried tomatoes. Simmer for 15 to 20 minutes, or until slightly thickened.

5. Divide the lentil mixture evenly among the tortillas. Roll and enjoy!

Makes 4 servings. Per serving: *331 calories, 19 g protein, 61 g carbs (13 g fiber, 9 g sugars), 5 g fat, 0 mg cholesterol, 787 mg sodium*

Tackle Box Trout

2 **farmed rainbow trout fillets (5 to 6 oz each)**

1 **lemon, thinly sliced**

1 **Tbsp + 2 tsp extra-virgin olive oil**

sprigs of fresh basil, parsley, chervil, or lovage

kosher salt and freshly ground pepper, to taste

2 **cups Swiss chard, chopped**

1. Preheat the grill to medium heat, or preheat oven to 425°F. Place each fillet, skin side down, on a square of heavy-duty aluminum foil. Top each with lemon slices, 1 teaspoon of oil, and a few herb sprigs. Season lightly with salt and pepper. Fold and seal the edges of the foil to create a tent above the fillets.

2. Place packets on the grill rack (if using an oven, place on a large baking sheet) and cook, lid down, 10 to 12 minutes.

3. While the fish is cooking, sauté Swiss chard in the remaining 1 tablespoon olive oil.

4. When fish fillets are opaque, flaky, and just cooked through, remove them from heat. Let them rest for 2 minutes before serving with the chard.

Makes 2 servings. Per serving: *185 calories, 20 g protein, 1 g carbs (0 g fiber, 0 g sugars), 11 g fat, 56 mg cholesterol, 312 mg sodium*

Colonel Mustard's Pork Chops

1   Tbsp maple syrup
1   Tbsp Dijon mustard
1   tsp olive oil
1   small clove garlic, crushed
     salt and ground black pepper, to taste
2   bone-in pork chops

1. Preheat a cast-iron skillet to medium-high.

2. In a small bowl, stir together the syrup, mustard, oil, garlic, salt, and pepper.

3. Place the pork chops and mustard mixture inside a large resealable plastic bag, then shake thoroughly to coat the chops.

4. Place the chops on the skillet, cooking 3 to 4 minutes per side. In the last minute of cooking, pour the remaining mustard mixture onto the chops.

Makes 2 servings. Per serving: *282 calories, 39 g protein, 9 g carbs (0 g fiber, 6 g sugars), 9 g fat, 123 mg cholesterol, 575 mg sodium*